MAKING THE
ANTIDEPRESSANT
DECISION

Also by Carol Ann Turkington

The Blood Thinner Cure
(with Kenneth R. Kensey, M.D.)

The Brain Encyclopedia

The Encyclopedia of Deafness and Hearing Disorders
(with Allen E. Sussman)

The Encyclopedia of Infectious Diseases
(with Bonnie Ashby, M.D.)

The Encyclopedia of Fertility and Infertility
(with Michael M. Alper)

The Encyclopedia of Memory and Memory Disorders
(with Richard Noll)

The Hearing Loss Sourcebook

Hepatitis C: The Silent Epidemic

The Home Health Guide to Poisons and Antidotes
(with Shirley Osterhout, M.D.)

The Hypericum Handbook: Nature's Antidepressant

Living with Hearing Loss (with Allen E. Sussman)

The Memory Sourcebook (with Joseph Harris)

Natural Cures for the Common Cold

The Perimenopause Sourcebook (with Susan Johnson)

Protect Yourself from Contaminated Food and Drink

Skin Deep: An A–Z of Skin and Skin Disorders
(with Jeffrey S. Dover, M.D.)

Stress Management for Busy People

12 Steps to a Better Memory

The Unofficial Guide to Women's Health
(with Susie J. Probst, M.D.)

MAKING THE ANTIDEPRESSANT DECISION

How to Choose the Right Treatment Option for You or Your Loved One

Carol Turkington and Eliot F. Kaplan, M.D.

Contemporary Books

Chicago   New York   San Francisco   Lisbon   London   Madrid   Mexico City
Milan   New Delhi   San Juan   Seoul   Singapore   Sydney   Toronto

Library of Congress Cataloging-in-Publication Data

Turkington, Carol.
    Making the antidepressant decision : how to choose the right treatment option for
you or your loved one / Carol Turkington, with Eliot F. Kaplan.
        p.   cm.
    ISBN 0-7373-0417-0
    1. Depression, Mental—Treatment.   2. Depression, Mental—Chemotherapy.
3. Psychopharmacology.   I. Kaplan, Eliot F.   II. Title.

    RC537 .T868   2001
    616.85'2706—dc21   2001032307

Contemporary Books

A Division of The McGraw-Hill Companies

Previously published as *Making the Prozac Decision* (1997)

1 2 3 4 5 6 7 8 9 0   DOC/DOC   0 9 8 7 6 5 4 3 2 1

ISBN 0-7373-0417-0

This book was set in ITC Galliard by Carolyn Wendt
Printed and bound by R. R. Donnelley—Crawfordsville

Cover design by Bill Stanton/Stanton Design
Cover illustration © George Schill/Stock Illustration Source

McGraw-Hill books are available at special quantity discounts to use as premiums and sales promotions, or for use
in corporate training programs. For more information, please write to the Director of Special Sales, Professional
Publishing, McGraw-Hill, Two Penn Plaza, New York, NY 10121-2298. Or contact your local bookstore.

"No one is capable of gratitude as one who has emerged from the kingdom of the night."

—*Elie Wiesel*

To my old friends Elaine and Jill, who have known the kingdom of the night.

—*Carol Ann Turkington*

To all those people thinking about pursuing treatment, as well as those currently in treatment for depression.

—*Eliot F. Kaplan, M.D.*

Contents

FOREWORD

I have been gratified by the positive response to *Making the Antidepressant Decision*. Shedding light on the appropriate use of antidepressants is the central focus of this book, and the prescription of antidepressant medication consumes an increasing proportion of the practicing psychiatrist's time and effort. With the increasing development of managed care in recent years, psychiatrists are called on less frequently to provide psychotherapy (now usually conducted by psychologists, social workers, and nurse psychotherapists) and more frequently to prescribe psychiatric drugs. My own practice is not immune to this trend.

There seems to be an increasing public acceptance of the "reality" of depression and the need for treatment. The selective serotonin reuptake inhibitors (SSRIs) are widely prescribed by primary care physicians as well as psychiatrists. I have seen an increase in interest and questions about alternative approaches as well—including acupuncture, Thought Field Therapy, Eye Movement Desensitization Reprocessing (EMDR), and herbal medications such as St. John's wort.

I completed my training in 1984, before the introduction of the newer antidepressants: the selective serotonin reuptake inhibitors (Prozac, Zoloft, Luvox, Celexa, and Paxil), Wellbutrin, and Effexor. Most of my career has been in the private practice of psychiatry, seeing outpatients in my office, working with patients in a 300-bed community hospital, treating patients on the mental health unit there, and doing consulting work with patients admitted medically. I have treated thousands of depressed patients (both male and female from their teens to their nineties), with symptoms ranging from mild adjustment problems to suicidal thoughts and/or psychosis. The work I have done is clinical, involving treatment rather than research or teaching.

My approach to treatment has typically started with patient education, including a summary of their situation, diagnosis, treatment options (with pros and cons), and prognosis. I try to help patients reach their goals, if that's feasible. I believe it's important to provide a trusting environment in which patients can discuss what is important to them. My approach is eclectic, using elements of insight, supportive and behavioral therapies, and antidepressant medication if needed.

It is important to realize that depression is a symptom of an illness, not a manifestation of moral or spiritual weakness. Depressive illness is akin to some medical problems with physiological bases that are affected by situational and temperamental factors such as hypertension, headache, diabetes mellitus, and irritable bowel syndrome. There are several types of depressive illness of varying severity, including adjustment disorder with depressed mood, dysthymia, major depressive episode, and bipolar disorder (manic-depressive illness). Before you embark on treatment for depression, it's important to have an evaluation to rule out any medical problems that could be causing or aggravating the depression.

It is worth considering what antidepressant medications do. They correct neurotransmitter problems in the brain that are associated with depression. About 80 percent of the time, they are extremely effective in helping with depression and the concomitant crying, sleep and appetite disturbances, suicidal ideas, feelings of hopelessness, concentration problems, lack of energy and interest, and so on. These medications work for as long as they're taken; they're a symptomatic treatment. The reason a person continues to do well after the antidepressant medication is stopped is that the depression has run its course.

Antidepressant medications work fairly quickly, sometimes within a few weeks, rather than the months that are typically needed in a purely psychotherapeutic approach. I've seen patients who have been in psychotherapy elsewhere for years without much benefit. When I've tried antidepressant medications in those patients, the results have often been excellent. Antidepressant medications can complement psychotherapy. The better a person feels, the more he or she can participate in the treatment. Patients with severe depression can be so preoccupied and withdrawn that they can't engage in psychotherapy at all until they've had some symptom relief.

It is also important to realize what antidepressant medications *don't* do. In my opinion, they do *not* change personality; they treat depression. Depression can cause withdrawal, poor self-esteem, timidity, quietness, and lack of enthusiasm. Treatment frees the person to be himself or herself. The depression may have persisted for years with an insidious onset, complicating and obscuring the pervasiveness of the symptoms. Antidepressant medications are not addictive. Antidepressant medications do not turn people into zombies. Antidepressant medications do not cure depression. They are part of a treatment regimen.

While the prescription of antidepressant medication in 2001 is as much art as science, I believe that any physician prescribing these drugs should have an organized, step-by-step approach should the first (or second or third) medication fail to help. Such an approach is often called a *decision tree.*

Typically, the first drug of choice to treat depression is an SSRI such as Prozac, Zoloft, Luvox, Celexa, or Paxil; if that doesn't relieve the person's depression, following is how I would proceed to the next drug of choice, and the next, and so on along my own decision tree:

Step 1. SSRI: Either Prozac, Zoloft, Luvox, Celexa, or Paxil

Step 2. *If no sexual dysfunction:*
different SSRI than above three

If there is sexual dysfunction:
with anxiety—Serzone
without anxiety—Wellbutrin

Step 3. Effexor

Step 4. Remeron

Step 5. tricyclic antidepressant (Pamelor or Norpramin)

Step 6. monoamine oxidase inhibitor (Nardil or Parnate)

Step 7. herbal preparation (St. John's wort)

Step 8. *Very rarely:*
electroconvulsive treatment (ECT)

A patient who responds partially to one of the above antidepressants often benefits from the addition of another drug, such as BuSpar, lithium, or Ritalin, for example. Obviously, there are exceptions and deviations from the decision tree—that's where the art comes in.

A commonly asked question is "How long should I take this antidepressant?" For a major depressive episode, the medication is typically continued for about six months before a reduction is tried. If the symptoms recur, the original dosage is resumed. For a dysthymia, a mild but persistent form of depression, the reduction is tried after a year. I warn patients that the depression may reappear in the future. If that happens, early resumption of treatment is advisable. Typically, restarting a medication that worked in the past will prove successful. In rare situations, the recommendation is lifelong medication.

What's important for you to understand is that the treatment of depression is typically *very* successful—*if* you keep trying if the first drug combination doesn't work. Sometimes persistence is needed.

In summary, depressive illnesses deserve prompt, aggressive therapy. Without treatment, depression can end in suicide. At the very least, depression affects the quality of life of those suffering from it.

To the millions of people plagued by depression: I encourage you to take the first step by getting a thorough psychiatric evaluation. You and your psychiatrist can work together to make the decisions that are best for you. For most, treatment does work.

—*Eliot F. Kaplan, M.D.*

ACKNOWLEDGMENTS

This book would not have been possible without the cooperation of countless women and men whose generosity of spirit contributed to *Making the Antidepressant Decision*. My heartfelt thanks to these people who so willingly shared their deeply personal stories of depression so that others might learn from their experiences. Special thanks for valuable referrals given by Dr. Jack Sturgis, Gail Novick, Jill Selleck, Elaine Bernarding and Barbara Turkington, and to Ross, for all the inside scoops.

Thanks also to a wide variety of psychiatric experts who have discussed their personal approach to antidepressant therapy, and to the staffs of the American Psychological Association, American Psychiatric Association, the National Institutes of Health, and the medical libraries of the National Library of Medicine, Hershey Medical Center, and the University of Pennsylvania Medical Center. Thanks also to Steve Berchem at Pharmaceutical Research and Manufacturers of America and to staffers at Eli Lilly, Astra USA, Bristol-Myers, Burroughs Wellcome, Ciba-Geigy, Hoffmann-LaRoche, Pfizer, SmithKline Beecham, and Solvay Pharmaceuticals.

Finally, my thanks to my agent Bert Holtje, for all his help; to Peter Hoffman for tireless support and terrific editing; and most of all, to Michael and to Kara, who have so generously shared me with my computer.

—*Carol Ann Turkington*

I would like to thank Roseann, my best friend and wife (and an excellent nurse psychotherapist), for her love and support.

I appreciate the thorough, broad-based training that I had at Jefferson Medical College and then in my psychiatry residency at Thomas Jefferson University Hospital in Philadelphia, which helped me to become the psychiatrist I am today.

I would like to thank my children, Melanie and Jason, for their love and patience while I worked on this book.

—*Eliot F. Kaplan, M.D.*

Introduction

"I was depressed my entire life. I kept going to doctors and telling them I didn't feel right. I felt icky. Crummy. Yucky. Once I started taking antidepressants, I realized I never felt like this in my entire life. It's called well-being."

—Susan, 38

To be depressed is to live with a sense of nothingness. People who are depressed say they feel numb, they feel empty, they feel invisible. Incredibly, two out of every eight Americans live their lives teetering on the edge of such an abyss, without any expectation that things will ever get better.

Who are they? They're people like Violet, a 38-year-old South Carolina nurse who developed depression following a liver transplant. "When I became depressed, I had no emotions at all," she recalls. "I always delighted at spring in South Carolina. But when I was depressed, I could look at the blooms and know it was beautiful, *but I had no sensory enjoyment of it.* I had my cat for 10 years, but when she died I didn't feel anything. Even as I was burying her, I felt nothing."

For four months, Violet hid her depression. "I really thought it was my fault," she says. "I thought my depression was an inappropriate response to receiving a life-saving organ. It wasn't okay to be feeling this way." When she finally confessed her depression to a psychiatrist, she was immediately given Prozac.

Within a few weeks, her depression began to lift. "It wasn't that I was suddenly effusive," Violet recalls. "I just started *feeling* again. Then one day, I came back from the store with extra supplies of dishwashing detergent and toothpaste, and I realized I was going to live. On a very deep level, I knew I would be washing my dishes and brushing my teeth two weeks from now. To me, it was a sign that I was getting better."

Perhaps you know someone like Violet—or maybe you feel this way yourself. You may have heard glowing reports about Prozac or one of the other new drugs in this class—Zoloft, Paxil, Celexa, or Luvox.

Perhaps you've heard rumors of drug-induced violence, the accusations that these drugs may change not just how you feel but *who you are.*

Are these drugs some sort of new salvation for depressed people, or is there a price to pay for the elimination of misery? Some experts warn that these medications are fads that promise to pave the way to nirvana for nondepressed people.

Psychiatrist Richard Metzner is a UCLA associate professor of psychiatry who says he's prescribed Prozac for hundreds of patients and doesn't know of one who's experienced the kind of miraculous personality change that was discussed on talk shows and in the media. The notion of Prozac as a personality pill was characterized by psychiatrist Peter Kramer, author of the best-seller *Listening to Prozac*, who described its effects as cosmetic, not therapeutic. Metzner argued that Prozac returns the working of the chemical composition of the brain to normal—and that, he said, is far from cosmetic.

Sorting out the pros and cons of antidepressant therapy can be a daunting task. But given the numbers of Americans currently taking these drugs, it's an important one. *Making the Antidepressant Decision* provides the latest information on antidepressants and the possible risks and benefits of these drugs. You'll also hear from men and women who've used all sorts of medications, some of which worked and some of which didn't.

Making the Antidepressant Decision can help you understand what depression is and how it can be treated. Sidebars provide additional information on side effects and possible drug interactions. You'll learn how to handle depression, how to tell if someone's depressed or suicidal, and how to join an experimental antidepressant study.

Making the Antidepressant Decision will help you understand the differences between antidepressants, as well as the potential side effects, problems, and benefits of each drug. You'll also find an extensive list of organizations to contact for further information.

Antidepressant therapy involves complex medical decisions between you and your doctor. It's vital that you understand the benefits and risks of this type of treatment because depression is not a simple problem. If you get a prescription for an antidepressant and it's just not helping or you can't tolerate the side effects, be honest about it. You need to form a working alliance with your doctor and to understand that there is no shame in getting help. If you're not getting relief with a particular antidepressant, it's not your fault.

There's no miracle antidepressant that works for everybody, every time. If you're taking an antidepressant drug now, is it the best choice for you? Do you fully understand the side effects of the drugs you're taking? If one antidepressant isn't working, is your doctor willing to find one that does?

"If the first drug doesn't work, don't give up," cautions psychiatrist Andy Myerson of North Carolina. "You need to go to a psychiatrist who won't judge you. Some doctors tend to say, 'If you don't get better, it's your fault.' But I've found that it's important to keep trying different antidepressants, because the tenth drug might work. Keep calling your doctor if you can't stand the side effects. If he or she won't help you, go to someone else."

1 WHAT IS DEPRESSION?

> *"When I was a teenager, it was as if one day a curtain dropped and I fell into the deepest, darkest abyss. That's what I've been battling for more than 25 years. My depression interfered with every conceivable part of my life."*
>
> —*Alison, 47*

Eleanor, 40, is a bright, attractive, well-educated Denver stockbroker who has struggled with feelings of overwhelming sadness for at least 25 years. "I can't remember when I wasn't depressed," she says today. Although her depression probably began in childhood, it was in college that she realized something was very wrong.

"I tried Rolfing, transactional analysis, meditation. I cut out coffee, smoking, and alcohol. I went on vegetarian diets, juice diets, and fasts. I kept trying all these alternative therapies because I thought that something should help the way I felt."

How she felt, she says, was miserable. "My body ached, the way you feel right before you get the flu—lethargic and hurting. That's why I smoked dope and drank alcohol; I was trying anything to feel better. But nothing worked." Then, in her mid-thirties Eleanor was injured in a car accident, and her depression deepened.

"I cried all day long. I would cry at every TV show—even 'Gunsmoke' and 'I Love Lucy'," she recalls. "I kept asking doctors why I was so depressed." Eleanor's psychologist finally became angry: "One day she snapped at me," Eleanor recalls, "and she said, 'Do you want me to send you to a psychiatrist so you can *take pills?*' She said it as if taking pills was a moral failure."

After another six months of fruitless talk therapy, Eleanor finally did go to see a psychiatrist, who did indeed prescribe an antidepressant for her depression—one of the most serious cases he said he'd ever seen. After her doctor tried three or four different medications, Eleanor's depression finally responded to a combination of Paxil and lithium.

"I feel as if I've been ripped off my entire life because I was depressed for so long," Eleanor says. "Now I have my sense of humor back. I feel great. I feel *normal.*"

Many people have stories similar to Eleanor's. Depression is far more common than most people realize: Two out of every 10 of us are clinically depressed. As many as 23 percent of all adult women have had one major depressive episode in their lifetime.

The tragedy is that although so many people are struggling silently with crushing misery, so few get help. There are 100,000 Eleanors in this country who haven't been correctly diagnosed and who aren't receiving treatment that could mean the difference between life and death.

Even today, too many Americans are intolerant of any type of mental illness—*especially* depression, which is often dismissed as some sort of moral failure. In a recent poll by the National Institute of Mental Health, nearly half of all respondents stated that depression was a "personal weakness"—certainly not a health problem.

It was precisely this intolerance that drove a noted Pennsylvania jurist to try to cover up his depression by having his employees fill his Prozac prescriptions—a felony. He finally confessed to the subterfuge because he said being labeled a drug trafficker was worse than being branded "depressed."

Depression has touched the lives of the most successful and brilliant men and women of our time. Sylvia Plath, Dick Cavett, Georgia O'Keeffe, Mark Twain, Virginia Woolf, and Abraham Lincoln all wrestled with depression.

"I felt a kind of numbness, an enervation," recalls William Styron in his book *Darkness Visible: A Memoir of Madness,* an account of his herculean struggle with major depression. "Mysteriously and in ways that are totally remote from normal experience, the gray drizzle of horror induced by depression takes on the quality of physical pain."

Is It the Blues—or Depression?

Of course, we all feel a little sad, dejected, or blue now and then. Fleeting unhappiness may briefly cloud your horizon after you lose a job, break up with your lover, or move to a new town. The profound mourning following the death of a loved one may last for several months—a completely normal response to a deeply felt emotional loss. The key difference between sad feelings and a true major depression is that sad feelings eventually pass, according to Douglas Jacobs, a Harvard Medical School psychiatrist who has devised national screening programs for depression.

"There were lots of times when I felt blue or sad," notes Sarah, 42, a North Carolina secretary. "Even when my divorce came through and my father died three weeks later, I managed to work through my sad feelings. But when I experienced major depression, it was very different.

"Before that, I had no idea what true depression was all about," Sarah explains. "Now there is a big 'D' and a little 'd' for me. Whenever people say that depression isn't a real mental disease, I find myself explaining just how terrible it can be."

As Sarah discovered, major depression is far more persistent than simple sadness. It descends as a sort of psychic cloud, numbing the soul with the conviction that the bleak outlook *will never change*. It interferes with sleep, appetite, sexual interest, self-image, and attitude. If you suffer from major depression, you can't just "snap out of it." And these dreadful feelings can last for weeks, months, or even years.

It is a disorder that costs this country dearly. The federal government estimates the cost of all types of depression is $43.7 billion each year—$12.4 billion in medical, psychiatric, and drug costs; $7.5 billion in depression-related suicide; and $23.8 billion in work absenteeism and lost productivity.

While effective therapy for depression has been available for decades, the condition is seriously undertreated in the United States, according to a panel of mental health experts reporting in the February 1997 *Journal of the American Medical Association*. This may either be due to the fact that doctors don't have the necessary training to effectively treat depression or because they may not view the condition seriously enough.

"There is still an enormous gap between our knowledge about the correct diagnosis and treatment of depression and the actual treatment that is being received in this country," wrote the panel led by psychiatrist Robert M. A. Hirschfield, M.D., at the University of Texas at Galveston.

Some studies have shown that only 1 in 10 Americans with depression get adequate treatment. When left untreated, depression can interfere with personal relationships and job performance and can increase your risk for other illnesses, according to a panel organized by the National Depressive and Manic Depressive Association. The number one cause of disability worldwide, depression is an increasing risk with age; it's expected to be the second leading cause of disease by the year 2020. In the United States, an estimated 6 million people are being actively treated for depression.

Major depression can be very hard to recognize, because it's a chronic, progressive disease. If you have major depression you may go into remission, but chances are that without treatment, it usually strikes again, more quickly and more powerfully than before.

Diagnosing Depression

A diagnosis may begin with a brief family history combined with a medical workup, including tests to rule out underactive thyroid, mononucleosis, anemia, diabetes, adrenal insufficiency, and hepatitis. Your doctor will want to know about any medications you've been taking, since a number of prescription drugs can cause depression (see box on page 32, "Drugs That Cause Depression"). While you're at it, you might also let your doctor know about any vitamins, herbal medicines, amino acids, diet supplements, or recreational drugs you have taken.

Major Depression

While symptoms differ from one person to the next, major depression is almost always characterized by general feelings of sadness and a total loss of pleasure in things that once brought you joy. You might also have sleep and eating problems or a sense of worthlessness. Perhaps you're no longer interested in sex, you're feeling apathetic, or you have suicidal thoughts.

According to the fourth edition of the *Diagnostic and Statistical Manual of Mental Disorders,* published by the American Psychiatric Association, a typical episode of a major depressive disorder lasts at least two weeks and includes most of the symptoms listed in the box, "Are You Depressed?"

Other common signs of depression may not be found in medical journals. "I ask patients if there are cobwebs in their house," says psychiatrist Andy Myerson, M.D. "If patients aren't bathing, if their house isn't clean, if they can't get out of bed—that's a good indication that they're depressed."

Many people in the midst of depression agree with him. "If I have to fight my way to the bathroom and I haven't opened my mail," Violet laughs, "I know I'm in trouble."

It is possible, however, to have a major depression and not feel particularly sorrowful, sad, or hurting. You may instead have eating problems or problems sleeping, remembering, concentrating, or making decisions. Only a mental health expert can diagnose a depression that is hiding as some of these symptoms.

ARE YOU DEPRESSED?

➤ Emotions: Do you feel ineffably sad or cry a great deal?

➤ Appetite/weight: Have you gained or lost weight? Do you binge or overeat?

➤ Sleep: Do you have chronic insomnia or excessive sleepiness? Are you tired all the time, regardless of how much sleep you get?

➤ Anger: Do you experience outbursts of complaints or shouting? Have you been feeling resentful and angry?

➤ Outlook: Have you lost interest in hobbies or activities that you formerly enjoyed?

➤ Libido: Have you lost interest in sex?

➤ Self-esteem: Do you feel worthless, unattractive, inappropriately guilty?

➤ Concentration: Do you have a hard time concentrating? Are your thoughts muddy or foggy?

➤ Anxiety: Do you brood, have phobias, delusions, or fears?

➤ Restlessness: Do you have trouble sitting still?

➤ Muted affect: Do you have slow body movements and speech?

➤ Suicide: Have you thought you'd be better off dead?

Dysthymic Disorder

Not everyone gets depressed in the same way. If you have a major depression (known as "unipolar" or "clinical depression"), your feelings of misery may be interrupted by periods when you feel okay. On the other hand, if you have a chronic minor depression (now called "dysthymic disorder"), you'll feel mildly depressed all the time; this constant low-level depression can last for years at a stretch. You may even have both types of depression at the same time.

"My problem with dysthymic disorder was characterized by fatigue," says Aguri, a 45-year-old psychologist who lives in New York. "By the afternoon, I became very tired and less clear in my thinking; I had to take a nap every afternoon or I couldn't work in the evening." Burdened by mounting job responsibilities, he finally sought help from his physician, who suggested the tricyclic Elavil. "It really helps," Aguri reports. "When I lower the dose or stop taking it, I can't sleep well and I get very tired. It helps improve my energy level."

Called depressive neurosis in the 1950s and depressive personality in the 1970s, dysthymic disorder is a persistent mild type of depression affecting as many as 3 million people. In order to be diagnosed with dysthymic disorder, you must have been depressed during most of the past two years, with at least two of the following six symptoms:

➤ Low self-esteem

➤ Poor appetite or overeating

➤ Insomnia or increased sleeping

➤ Difficulty concentrating or making decisions

➤ Hopelessness

➤ Fatigue or low energy

This type of mild depression can be misdiagnosed as borderline personality disorder, which in itself does not respond to antidepressants. Dysthymic disorder, however, can be treated with antidepressants.

Double Depression

If you've been struggling with a long-term dysthymic disorder and suddenly experience a major depression, your psychiatrist will diagnose a "double depression." Many doctors have successfully used the new SSRIs, including Prozac, in such cases to treat the dysthymic disorder and prevent the return of major depression. Controlling this combination of depressions may require a slightly higher dosage.

Atypical Depression

If you find that you continually crave sleep, food, or sex over a period of two weeks or more, you may be developing what's called "atypical depression."

Most depressed people don't sleep or eat enough, and many lose weight, but people with atypical depression *gain* weight and sleep too much. They're also anxious and extremely sensitive to their environment and to rejection.

Atypical depressions may be disguised as bulimia, anorexia, compulsive overeating, oversleeping, addictions, or impulsiveness. While some of these symptoms are also found in major depression, they aren't as severe and don't last as long. If you have an atypical depression, you may feel that your phobias, symptoms, or hysterical feelings are more troublesome than your depression, but, in fact it's the depression that causes these symptoms.

Experts don't know why atypical depression appears in many ways as the polar opposite of major depression or why it's more common in women than in men. But we do know that without treatment, the symptoms will probably get worse. In the past, patients like this responded best to one of the MAOIs; today, the SSRIs (including Prozac) appear to be just as effective.

Subclinical Depression

If you have only two or three symptoms of depression as opposed to five or more, your doctor may diagnose a "subclinical depression." If you're so diagnosed, it is likely that you've never sought mental health treatment, since you can probably function fairly well despite low self-confidence, timidity, lack of interest, sadness, emptiness, or fatigue. Psychotherapy alone may not solve these problems if they are of long standing, but many people with subclinical depression respond well to Prozac or another SSRI in conjunction with psychotherapy.

Other Forms of Depression

The symptoms of psychotic depression may include delusions of guilt, serious medical illness, and a feeling of deserving punishment for imagined mistakes. There may also be auditory hallucinations or other delusions. The melancholic type of depression includes lack of the ability to have even fleeting good feelings, a worsening of mood in the morning, early morning awakening (between three and four o'clock), more than 5 percent weight loss per month, agitation or lethargy, and loss of interest in all activities.

Manic-Depression (Bipolar Disorder)

A person with manic-depression suffers through alternating periods of severe depression and manic "highs" that can be severe enough to require hospitalization. When you experience a manic phase, you may be elated, irritable, or paranoid—you're probably hyperactive, concentrating on all sorts of risky activities. During this phase, you might talk very quickly and loudly, switching from one topic to another. You might go for days without rest, spend money you don't have, become promiscuous, eat and drink too much, or begin to think you can conquer the world. You might entice others to join you in wild business schemes. Eventually, you may begin to have serious delusions about your own abilities.

But after days or weeks of feeling all-powerful, suddenly you come crashing to earth in a profound depression that leaves you feeling defeated and doomed. The world that just yesterday was bright and full of promise is today a bleak and gray disaster.

John was a successful pediatrician when he was diagnosed with manic-depression in his early thirties. For some years, his behavior had become increasingly erratic; periods of wild enthusiasm would be followed by months of black despair during which he dragged himself through seemingly endless days and sleepless nights. During one manic phase, he became obsessed with a pyramid scheme for selling auto products. Soon his entire home was converted into a warehouse, and he listened to motivational tapes produced by company executives at all hours of the day and night. His obsession soon drove him to harangue patients and colleagues to join him in selling the products or listening to the tapes. Not until both his practice and his professional reputation were in serious jeopardy was he induced to seek treatment.

Manic-depression can strike anyone. Some of history's most creative individuals are now believed to have been manic-depressives; some even created masterpieces during a manic phase.

Like other forms of depression, manic-depression appears to be caused by a biochemical imbalance in the brain that requires a combined treatment of medications (usually lithium) and therapy. While there is strong evidence that manic-depression has a genetic component, just because a sister, brother, or parent has the disease doesn't mean you're doomed to follow the same path. In many cases, too much stress trips a biological vulnerability mechanism and pushes a person into manic-depression.

Obsessive-Compulsive Disorder

People with this disorder become obsessed with certain thoughts (obsessions) and bogged down with repetitive activities (compulsions) such as washing their hands or rechecking doors and windows. Often, the compulsions are a way to ease the anxiety that arises from the obsessive thoughts.

If you have OCD, you may be fearful about dirt, disease, or toxic chemicals, or you may need to count, align, check, or apologize constantly.

People with OCD aren't out of touch with reality. They *know* their behavior isn't reasonable, and about a third are so upset about their problems that they become clinically depressed.

OCD is often treated successfully using a number of different antidepressants, some of which are specifically approved by the FDA for the treatment of OCD. Usually patients who respond best are those who combine drug therapy with some type of counseling.

Panic Disorder

This condition begins with a sudden feeling of intense doom or apprehension and brings with it a host of physical symptoms including heart palpitations, shortness of breath, dizziness, weakness, sweating, choking, nausea, and tingling. Panic disorder is often misdiagnosed as a respiratory or cardiac problem. People with this problem often link their attacks of panic to the specific place where it occurred, which is why someone who has a panic attack in an elevator will begin to avoid all elevators. Medications usually used to treat panic attacks include either the tricyclics or the SSRIs. Behavior modification combined with relaxation therapy can be an extremely important part of treatment as well.

Suicide Risk

Because the primary risk of depression is suicide, a good diagnosis and effective treatment are critical. At least 80 percent of suicides never got that treatment (see box on page 14, "Warning Signs of Potential Suicide").

Suicide is the eighth leading cause of death in this country—and the second leading cause of death among teenagers. It's estimated that 30,000 Americans kill themselves each year, and at least 10 times that number

---

WARNING SIGNS OF POTENTIAL SUICIDE

A person thinking about suicide may show one or more of the following symptoms, but these are only guidelines. There is no single "typical" suicide profile. A person showing suicidal signs should be encouraged to seek professional help as soon as possible. Start by calling local suicide hotlines or a local psychiatrist or psychologist immediately.

➤ Suicide threats: The widespread belief that people who threaten suicide never follow through on that threat is not true.
➤ Withdrawal: An overwhelming urge to be alone or an unwillingness to communicate, withdrawing into a shell. Trouble with grades or on the job can signal such a retreat.
➤ Life crisis: Death, divorce, job loss, or accident can trigger suicide in a deeply depressed person.
➤ Behavior change: Changes in appearance, energy, or attitude.
➤ Aggression: Sudden interest in dangerous pursuits, sports, or unsafe sexual practices.
➤ Moodiness: Sudden calm after severe depression may indicate a person has chosen suicide as a solution to problems.
➤ Gift-giving: Sudden bequeathing of treasured possessions.

make unsuccessful attempts. The problem is particularly troubling among the young: five teenagers a day commit suicide in the United States. Although the rate among adolescents tripled from 1957 to 1987, it stabilized in the late 1980s. For every teenager who commits suicide, about 200 try. Moreover, research shows that those who have ever been hospitalized for depression have a 15 percent higher risk for suicide.

While suicide is more common among men, women make four times as many attempts. It's most prevalent among the elderly, those without a significant partner in their lives, those with chronic medical problems, and those with mood disorders.

Most people who are seriously depressed admit to having suicidal thoughts at some point, and many act on those thoughts. In fact, a depressed person is 35 times more likely to commit suicide.

Causes of Depression

The majority of experts agree that depression has no one specific cause. Instead, it's the result of a collision between genetics, biochemistry, and psychological factors.

Neurotransmitters

The physiological basis of depression can be found in nerve cells in the part of the brain responsible for human emotions centered in the hypothalamus, a cherry-size structure that controls basic functions such as thirst, hunger, sleep, sexual desire, and body temperature. Each nerve cell in your brain is separated by tiny gaps; neurotransmitters communicate by ferrying messages across these gaps to a "receptor" on the other side. Each neurotransmitter has a special shape that helps it fit exactly into a corresponding receptor like a key in an ignition switch. When the neurotransmitter "key" is inserted into its matching receptor's "ignition," the cell fires and sends the message on its way. Once the message is sent, the neurotransmitter is either absorbed into the cell or burned up by enzymes patrolling the gaps.

When the levels of these neurotransmitters are abnormally low, messages can't get across the gaps, and communication in the brain slows down. It appears that depression occurs if you don't have enough of these neurotransmitters circulating in your brain or if your neurotransmitters can't fit into the receptors for some reason.

While there are as many as 100 different kinds of neurotransmitters, norepinephrine, serotonin, and dopamine seem to be of particular importance in depression. The pathways for these neurotransmitters reach deep into many of the parts of the brain responsible for functions that are affected in depression—sleep, appetite, mood, and sexual interest.

Scientists aren't sure whether depression is directly related to abnormal levels of these transmitters, or whether these neurotransmitters affect yet another neurotransmitter that's even more directly involved in depression. But it is clear that neurotransmitters are related to depression because medications that boost levels of these neurotransmitters also ease depression. Yet some of the newer antidepressants don't affect the levels of all these neurotransmitters, though they still relieve depression.

And other drugs (such as cocaine) that *do* interfere with neurotransmitter levels *don't* affect depression.

And here's the knottiest puzzle of all: Antidepressants can raise your neurotransmitter levels almost immediately, but your depression won't lift until weeks after drug therapy has begun. Depression appears to be far more than a simple problem with the amount of neurotransmitters in the synaptic cleft. Instead, it is probably influenced by a complex interplay of receptor "ignition" responses and the release of the neurotransmitter "keys." It also seems to depend not just on the *number* of neurotransmitter keys but on the *quality* and *availability* of the receptor ignitions.

Antidepressants appear to make certain receptors unreachable, which may explain the antidepressants' lag time. The inaccessibility of these receptors may trigger an increase in the production of neurotransmitters. These changes don't happen right after antidepressant treatment begins; they can take up to several weeks. This receptor change has been reported in almost all antidepressant drug treatment and also in electroconvulsive therapy.

Loss and Trauma

Most cases of depression seem to be triggered by a serious loss or unpleasant experience that pushes a person who may be genetically or psychologically susceptible into a depressive abyss.

That's what happened to Rod, 31, when his mother—his last surviving relative—suddenly died. Rod came from a troubled family dogged by alcoholism and depression.

When his long-suffering mother finally succumbed to a heart attack, Rod's world fell apart, and he entered a downward spiral of ever-deepening depression.

"Everything seemed gray and muffled," he recalled, "as if it were wrapped in cotton wool. Nothing had any color. Food had no taste. I couldn't sleep at night, and I'd stumble through my work."

In a study of 680 pairs of female twins, recent stress (a divorce, illness, bereavement, or legal problem) was the best predictor of depression. Other studies have found that as many as 86 percent of major depressions were set off by a life crisis.

At other times, a depressive disorder may seem to come out of the blue. It may be triggered by a physical illness, or it could be associated with hormonal changes after childbirth or during menopause. Some people become depressed after taking certain drugs (such as birth control pills, steroids, or sleeping pills).

That was the case with Cathy, whose serious manic-depression was triggered by massive doses of prednisone following a transplant operation.

"I was overdosed on prednisone," she reports, "and it made me feel terrible. I was a zombie."

Hormones

For some time, scientists have noticed that depression and problems with hormone regulation appear to go hand in hand. This link isn't really surprising, since hormones affect neurotransmitter activity, and neurotransmitters affect the timing and release of hormones. You may have noticed that depression tends to crop up during events related to reproduction (menstruation, ovulation, pregnancy, and menopause). Altered hormone levels during these times can affect mood-regulating neurotransmitters, but just how they accomplish this isn't clear.

PMS and Depression

Premenstrual syndrome (PMS) is usually associated with depression, irritability, exhaustion, sore breasts, bloating, and crying spells and affects most women in their twenties and thirties. Between 20 and 80 percent of women have some form of this problem, but according to the American Psychological Association Task Force on Women and Depression, only 5 percent experience significant discomfort and need professional treatment.

"I didn't have to look at a calendar to know when my period was due," confessed Kathy, 33, who suffers from premenstrual syndrome. "I'd start getting cranky and irritable a few days before my period, and then I'd get depressed. I'd snap at my family, and some days I just stayed in bed because I couldn't face the world. Then as soon as my period was over, I'd be perky as ever."

A woman's menstrual cycle is regulated by complex interactions between neurotransmitters (serotonin, dopamine, and norepinephrine), pituitary hormones, and ovarian hormones. We don't yet know exactly how the ovarian hormones interact with neurotransmitters or why the result varies so widely from one woman to the next, but it may have something to do with genetics. Your brain's ability to regulate neurotransmitters is strongly influenced by heredity.

Recent research at the University of California at San Diego found that some women who are depressed as a result of PMS have lower amounts of a brain chemical called melatonin when they sleep. Melatonin is released by the pineal gland to induce sleep and regulate circadian rhythms. Experts believe melatonin may suppress mood and mental quickness.

In fact, recent research has isolated serotonin as a possible culprit in PMS. In the late 1980s, several studies revealed that women who had PMS had lower serotonin levels right before their periods than did women who don't have PMS.

There may also be a link between serotonin levels, carbohydrate cravings, and PMS, according to similar studies at the Massachusetts Institute of Technology by neuroscientist Richard Wurtman and Judith Wurtman, a cell biologist and nutritionist. They have found that depression, carbohydrate craving, and a few other PMS symptoms can be relieved by the drug D-fenfluramine, which affects serotonin.

If you experience one week during the month when you don't feel normal, you may be diagnosed as having PMS; if your negative emotions occur all month long but are aggravated premenstrually, your problem might more correctly be diagnosed as a mood disorder.

While there are no well-established treatments that work consistently for PMS, many doctors are now using antidepressants to treat severe cases; both Prozac and the tricyclic nortriptyline have been reported to be of particular benefit to women with severe symptoms. Lithium has also been used successfully in certain types of PMS.

"We use [Prozac] for a great number of women with PMS, and the results are wonderful," reports one psychiatric nurse, who is certified to treat patients in practice with a psychiatrist. "You'd be surprised at how well it works for all the symptoms of PMS."

Try keeping a daily rating scale for several months. It's the best way to establish a link between your mood and your periods.

Of course, it could also be true that many women have mild depressions that respond well to antidepressants; once their depression is treated, the PMS-like symptoms disappear.

It's also important to realize that some cases of PMS may actually be an undiagnosed depression. In one study, two-thirds of the women with a history of major depression experienced more symptoms of PMS than those who were not chronically depressed. *Even after menopause,* many of these women still experienced PMS symptoms even though they didn't have the hormonal fluctuations that had supposedly triggered their PMS. This suggests that for *some* women, what appears to be PMS may in fact be an untreated depression.

Postpartum Depression

Up to 70 percent of all new mothers experience the "baby blues," a mild form of brief depression including crying spells, restlessness, feelings of unreality and confusion, depersonalization, guilt, and negative feelings toward both the husband and the child. Symptoms often fade within a week.

While the symptoms are well documented, scientists aren't sure whether these feelings are simply the result of a profound life-role change or a true metabolic disruption. However, it's clear that five days after delivery, the levels of estrogen and progesterone drop, and a burst of prolactin occurs. The lower the progesterone falls, the more likely it is that the mother will become depressed within 10 days after birth.

"I'd read about the baby blues, but I didn't really expect to feel sad," recalls Wanda, who had her first child at age 36. "I was always so perky. I've never been depressed in my life. But when I heard them wheeling my baby down the corridor to my room, my heart would actually sink. I felt terrible that instead of being thrilled at the prospect of seeing my baby, I just wanted to be left alone. I would lie in bed, and tears would roll down my cheeks for no apparent reason."

For Wanda, these feelings faded within a day or two. Other women aren't so lucky. One or 2 out of every 10 new mothers struggle with a more serious form of depression, which may last from six weeks to a year or more. These women worry constantly about their child's health and their own ability to have normal motherly feelings.

An even smaller number, just 0.01 to 0.02 percent, will develop postpartum psychosis between the third and fourteenth day after birth. This frightening development can appear quickly, ballooning from a moderate depression to delusions and hallucinations. In most cases, there is no prior history of depression and its occurrence seems to have nothing to do with other events in the woman's life. This high-risk condition must be treated with hospitalization, medication, and sometimes electro-shock therapy.

In general, women with a history of depression or manic-depression before pregnancy are at higher risk for developing postpartum depression.

Endocrine Disorders

There are several hormonal or endocrine diseases that may cause depression, including hypothyroidism (underactive thyroid gland), hyperthyroidism (overactive thyroid gland), Addison's disease (underactive adrenal gland), Cushing's syndrome (overactive adrenal gland), and either under- or overactivity of the parathyroid gland. Hormonal drugs (including birth control pills and steroids like cortisone and prednisone) may also cause depression.

Puberty

Puberty is the first of a series of reproduction-related events that appear to be strongly linked with depression. One study found that a woman's first major depressive episode was most likely to occur around the age of 13 or 14. A study of 1,500 New York youngsters found that severe depression affects 7 percent of all girls. But it's not just young women who suffer with depression at this age. Boys, too, can experience hormonal changes together with the problems of emerging identity, peer pressure, sexual issues, and increasing adult responsibilities, all combining to cause depression during adolescence.

Menopause and Depression

The idea that menopause and depression are interrelated phenomena is a hot potato widely disputed by many feminists. It's a fact that women go through hormonal changes during menopause, but scientists have been able to prove no clear-cut relationship between depression and menopause. Some experts believe that you may experience mood changes once your estrogen levels drop. Others suggest that low thyroid levels that often occur at this time may also influence depression.

The reduction of estrogen following menopause causes several problems, including osteoporosis (thinning of the bones), dryness and thinning of the vaginal walls, and an increased risk of heart disease. According to Dr. Ellen McGrath, chair of the American Psychological Association National Task Force on Women and Depression, women are probably more likely to be depressed over these physical changes than over the ending of menstruation.

Heart Disease and Depression

People who are depressed are more than twice as likely than others to develop high blood pressure, a major cause of heart disease, according to a study by the National Center for Health Statistics of the Centers for Disease Control and Prevention in Atlanta. Even intermediate levels of anxiety and depression were associated with a 60 percent greater likelihood of developing high blood pressure. While the link between depression and heart disease is found in both black and white patients, the risk is especially high for blacks.

Moreover, depressed people are four times more likely to have a heart attack than those with more positive states of mind, according to a study at the Johns Hopkins School of Hygiene and Public Health. In addition, people who are depressed are more likely to smoke, which is another known cause of heart disease.

Those with the highest levels of depression and anxiety were at greatest risk of developing high blood pressure. But even those with intermediate levels of anxiety and depression were also associated with hypertension.

Scientists suggest that the link between depression and heart disease may be due to biochemical changes that occur in depressed people, such as the secretion of stress hormones that weaken the immune system. Others believe depression leaves victims so unhappy that they neglect their health, forget to take medications like those that control high blood pressure, and thus become more vulnerable to heart attacks.

Migraines

The severe headache known as migraine, with accompanying symptoms of nausea, diarrhea, and visual disturbances, attacks about 8 million Americans, 75 percent of them women. They are believed to be linked to changes in the levels of estrogen and serotonin. Depression and stress also contribute to migraines.

Because of the suspected role of serotonin in migraine attacks, some doctors have been successful in treating them with a standard dose of one of the SSRIs—Prozac, Zoloft, Luvox, Celexa, or Paxil—which act exclusively on the serotonin system.

Heredity

Although there's no certain evidence that there is a single gene for depression, some families have an inherited vulnerability to depression (see box, "What Are Your Chances of Inheriting Depression?"). This is especially true in the case of manic-depression, where up to 50 percent of manic-depressives have at least one parent with the disorder.

"My father was an alcoholic and my brother is a manic-depressive," notes Eleanor. "It's not surprising that I have a problem with depression, too."

Science would tend to agree with her. A 1992 study of female identical twins found that if one twin has a major depression, the other (who shares all her genes) is

---

WHAT ARE YOUR CHANCES OF
INHERITING DEPRESSION?

➤ Relatives: Close relatives of depressed people have a 15 percent chance of inheriting major depression.

➤ Twins: If your identical twin is depressed, you're 67 percent more likely to be depressed.

➤ Substance abuse: If your depressed relatives abuse alcohol or drugs as a symptom of depression, you're 8 to 10 times more likely to do the same.

➤ Suicide: If you become depressed, you're much more vulnerable to suicide if a close relative has committed suicide.

➤ Women: Close female relatives of depressed women have a one in four chance of inheriting major depression and a 90 percent chance of having mild depression.

66 percent more likely to suffer from the same problem than are unrelated children. But among fraternal female twins (who share no more genes than nontwin sisters), one twin had only a 27 percent higher chance of sharing the other's depression.

Researchers have concluded that a person may not inherit depression solely as a result of one gene, the way you inherit hair or eye color. At most, say experts at the Medical College of Virginia, depression is probably only about 40 percent influenced by genes. People *can* inherit certain personality traits, collectively known as "depressive personality disorder," that may make them prone to depression. People with the disorder tend to be pessimistic and brooding, with an overly critical attitude toward themselves and others. It's also true that if you're seriously depressed, you may have a different sort of biochemistry, with high levels of the stress chemical cortisol and low levels of the calming neurotransmitters serotonin and norepinephrine.

Biological Rhythms

Your body's internal rhythm waxes and wanes with the ticking of the clock. For example, your body temperature rises during the day and falls during the evening. Biological rhythms such as hormone secretion and sleep-wake patterns have a 24-hour cycle and are called circadian rhythms.

It's not surprising that there may be a link between depression and biological rhythms, too. You may find your moods get better or worse in tune with the seasons or the time of day. Perhaps you've noticed that you tend to feel terrible in the morning but a bit better as the day wears on. Or maybe you feel worse and worse as the day proceeds.

"I was always at my worst during the morning," says Jennifer, 42, who takes Effexor to manage her depression. "Now, from 8:30 A.M. to 11 A.M., I'm feeling the way I wanted to feel for the last 20 years. I'm not weighted down by an ungodly weight."

Early-morning awakening is one of the hallmarks of clinical depression, and the continuing cycles of depression and mania are the hallmarks of manic-depression.

Seasonal Affective Disorder

The syndrome of winter depression, called seasonal affective disorder (SAD), is specifically related to changes in the length of daylight across the seasons. While its exact cause is unknown, the disorder has been linked to a malfunction in the body's biological clock that controls temperature and hormone production.

As many as 12 million Americans may suffer from this disorder, and up to 35 million others may experience milder forms. It's at least four times as common among women, usually beginning in the twenties and thirties (although it has been reported in some children and teenagers). Other estimates suggest that as many as half of all women in northern states experience pronounced winter depression, but very few receive the necessary treatment because their doctors don't know how to tell the difference between typical depressive symptoms and SAD.

"I start to feel depressed around November," says Anne, 40, a Pennsylvania probation officer. "It just keeps getting worse until the spring. It helps a little bit if I take naps, but what I really seem to need is the sunlight."

The pineal gland appears to be particularly important in the development of SAD. Nestling near the center of the brain, the gland processes information about light through special nerve pathways and releases the sleep-inducing hormone melatonin, also responsible for regulating circadian rhythms. Melatonin is produced in the dark and peaks during the winter. Experts believe it may suppress mood and mental quickness. Interestingly, manic-depressives are extremely sensitive to light, and exposure to it causes their melatonin levels to plummet.

Your body is regulated by some sort of biological clock that sets the pace for everyday rhythms of sleep, activity, temperature, and cortisol and melatonin release. Most people maintain a certain flexibility in this system, allowing them to synchronize this biological clock to environmental changes. But experts suspect that some people—perhaps those prone to depression—don't syn-chronize their clocks so easily. It could be that their internal clock is out of step with the world's 24-hour rhythm, so that melatonin is released too early (causing evening sleepiness and early-morning awakening) or too late (causing insomnia and trouble waking up).

In some cases, SAD eventually disappears, but in others it persists for a lifetime. The best treatment for this disorder is phototherapy—exposure to special types of bright light during the winter, 10 to 20 times brighter than normal indoor light for 15 to 30 minutes a day.

Animal research suggests that light therapy eases depression by helping to boost serotonin levels and mela-tonin. Researchers found that when hamsters were sub-jected to pulses of light, the levels of available serotonin in their brains rose. These findings, published in the January 1997 issue of *Nature*, also suggest that light therapy might help those with other disorders associated with low serotonin levels, such as obsessive-compulsive disorder.

SAD can be effectively and inexpensively treated in more than 75 percent of patients. However, it's important to get an accurate diagnosis and the right kind of light box to provide enough high-intensity light for a certain time each day (see box, "Where to Buy Light Fixtures to Treat Seasonal Affective Disorder"). After a few days of your sitting for several hours under special fluorescent lights, symptoms subside; they reappear if treatment stops. In general, patients must sit about three feet away from a bank of special lights of between six and eight fluorescent bulbs. Homemade versions can also be built. Ordinary room light is not bright enough to affect SAD. Photo-therapy is often more effective when begun before—not after—symptoms begin. Treatment should be under the supervision of an expert.

Because light therapy may be only partly successful in eradicating symptoms, treatment may be bolstered by the use of antidepressants. Antidepressants may be used alone instead of light therapy for people with SAD, but the two treatments are usually combined, which often means that lower doses of antidepressants are needed.

Don't be surprised if your doctor must adjust the dose of antidepressants with the changing seasons, increasing your dose as the days become shorter and decreasing it as the days lengthen.

More and more doctors are considering Prozac and the other SSRIs to be the drugs of choice for SAD, primarily because the serotonin system is believed to be part of the problem in this disorder. Desyrel has also been used successfully with SAD patients. Older antidepressants may also be beneficial, such as the tricyclics desipramine or imipramine. (Doctors often stay away from the more sedating tricyclics, such as amitriptyline and doxepin, since people with SAD tend to sleep too much as it is.)

A few depressed people with problems in their basic circadian rhythm appear to be helped—at least

---

WHERE TO BUY LIGHT FIXTURES TO TREAT
SEASONAL AFFECTIVE DISORDER

Bio-Brite, Inc.
7315 Wisconsin Avenue, Suite 1300W
Bethesda, MD 20814
(800-621-LITE)

The Sunbox Company
19217 Orbit Drive
Gaithersburg, MD 20879
(800-LITE-YOU) (800-548-3968)
www.sunboxco.com

Apollo Light Systems, Inc.
369 South Mountain Way Drive
Orem, UT 84058
(800-226-2370)
www.homehealthprovider.com/storefronts/apollo

Hughes Lighting Technologies
Yacht Club Drive
Lake Hopatcong, NJ 07849
(800-LIGHT-25) (973-663-1214)

temporarily—by staying up all night, then resuming their regular sleep-wake cycle, but others don't get any benefit from this treatment at all. While experts aren't sure why this works, they think it has something to do with shifting the basic circadian rhythm back to a normal 24-hour cycle. However, this treatment is experimental and should not be attempted by the patient without consultation with a physician.

Drugs That Cause Depression

A number of drugs now on the market may actually *cause* depression (see box, "Drugs That Cause Depression"). These include blood-pressure medications such as Catapres, Aldomet, and Inderal; drugs used to treat Parkinson's

---

DRUGS THAT CAUSE DEPRESSION

Drug-induced depression is more likely to be found in those who are genetically vulnerable to this disorder. The following drugs are known to cause depression in some people:

➤ Benzodiazepines
➤ Clonidine
➤ Cortisone-like steroids
➤ Digitalis
➤ Indomethacin
➤ Levodopa
➤ Methyldopa
➤ Oral contraceptives
➤ Phenothiazines (some)
➤ Reserpine

disease such as L-dopa and bromocriptine; diet pills and medicines prescribed for arthritis, ulcers, or seizures; and hormones like estrogen, progesterone, cortisol, and prednisone.

Moreover, some commonly prescribed tranquilizers such as Valium or Halcion, which are designed to calm you down, can on rare occasions stimulate violence, aggression, or depression. Styron described just such an occurrence in *Darkness Visible*. Because he suffered from insomnia as a result of his severe depression, he was given the sleeping pill Halcion. When he took inappropriately excessive doses, his depression appeared to get much worse. Styron blames the drug as a contributory factor in his downward spiral into profound depression.

Who Gets Depressed?

About 3 to 4 percent of Americans experience major depression. About 5 percent of Americans struggle with other forms of depression—dysthymic disorder (mild depression), chronic treatment-resistant depression, or depression caused by medical or other psychiatric disorders. Manic-depression affects another 1 to 2 percent.

If you've had one episode of major depression, you've got a 50 percent chance of having another bout—sometimes four or five episodes during a lifetime. Some people have recurrent depressive episodes separated by years of relatively good mental health. Others experience clusters of depression over a short period with a few glimpses of normal function in between. Unfortunately, as many as 35 percent of depressed people experience a chronic form of the condition that never fades away at all without treatment.

The problem appears to be on the increase. In the past century, each succeeding generation has experienced major depressions at earlier and earlier ages, and each generation that follows the next has a higher lifetime risk of experiencing the disorder.

Women and Depression

More than twice as many women as men are diagnosed with depression, although the reason why this occurs is still hotly debated. Today, experts predict that one in four women will experience a depressive episode sometime during her lifetime. Some experts blame physiology—heredity or hormonal imbalances. Others point to the different ways men and women learn to handle emotions, and the fact that health professionals more readily diagnose depression in women. Some blame social factors: a woman's lower economic status and susceptibility to abuse contribute to higher rates of depression. Physical and sexual abuse may also be major factors in women's depression, according to psychologist Ellen McGrath, author of *When Feeling Bad Is Good.* Experts have estimated that between 37 and 50 percent of women have had a significant experience of physical or sexual abuse before age 21. For many women, McGrath believes, depression may actually be the effects of post-traumatic stress syndrome.

Careful epidemiological studies have shown that the higher depressive ratio for women is *not* due to a woman's greater willingness to report depressive episodes; women really *do* get depressed at a higher rate.

The typical depressed woman is between 25 and 40, married, and raising children. Research does suggest that depression is most likely to be found at both ends of the economic spectrum—in professional women and those with low income, as well as in those with little personal support or substance abusers.

What many have trouble accepting is that some of a woman's vulnerability to depression may be biological. In fact, 1 out of every 10 women becomes seriously depressed after giving birth. Almost 90 percent report PMS symptoms, although they may not all be disturbed enough to qualify for a diagnosis of PMS. In women with PMS depression, serotonin levels are below those of women without PMS, and levels are lower before their periods than afterward.

Depression in Childhood

Most children will get a bit sad now and then when something goes wrong at home or school. When youngsters get the blues, their sad feelings should pass within a few days. If the depression deepens or continues longer than two weeks, it could indicate a more serious problem.

While most people think of depression as a disorder of adulthood, in fact it can appear at any age—even in infancy. Depressed children may become clingy, tired, listless, or anxious. They may refuse to go to school and may try to hurt themselves (banging their head against a wall, for example). They may lose interest in normal activities and start having problems in school. If the child's depression is severe enough, even a youngster no more than five or six may deliberately attempt suicide.

"I didn't want to live anymore," whispered one five-year-old boy as he lay dying after darting in front of a truck because he said he felt unloved.

A 1982 study of 3,000 children found that almost 15 percent of them had symptoms of depression; the same study found that by age 15, one out of five children were depressed.

The average length of depression in childhood is about seven months, but the younger the child, the more serious the prognosis. Odds are great that a child who has experienced one major depression will have another episode.

If you take your child to the doctor because of your concern about depression, the doctor will probably first take a complete medical history, focusing on the child's feelings, psychological traits, and social background. The visit should include a thorough physical exam to rule out underlying physical disorders.

In recent years, more and more doctors have begun to realize that youngsters can suffer from a wide variety of mood disorders and that they can be just as sick as any adult. As a result, the use of antidepressants and lithium in childhood has become much more common.

Indeed, medication may be an effective part of the treatment for several psychiatric disorders in childhood and adolescence, according to the American Academy of Child and Adolescent Psychiatry. If your doctor recommends medication for your child, he or she should be experienced in the treatment of psychiatric illnesses and should fully explain the reasons for the recommended drug, its benefits, side effects, and alternatives.

Parents must realize that medication should not be used alone but as part of a comprehensive treatment plan that usually includes some type of psychotherapy. In addition, your doctor should provide ongoing evaluation. When prescribed appropriately by an experienced psychiatrist, medication may help children and teenagers with psychiatric disorders feel better.

Psychiatric medication may be prescribed for a number of problems, including:

➤ *Depression:* lasting feelings of sadness, helplessness, hopelessness, unworthiness and guilt, inability to feel pleasure, declining school work, changes in sleeping or eating

➤ *Eating disorder:* either anorexia nervosa or bulimia or a combination of the two

➤ *Manic-depression* (bipolar disorder): periods of depression alternating with manic periods, including irritability, happy moods, excessive energy, behavior problems, staying up late at night, and grand plans

When a child is diagnosed with a full-blown major depression, an antidepressant such as imipramine or an SSRI may be considered in order to bring the child out of the depression, thereby avoiding harming the child's emotional growth and relationships.

Most experts think that children who have one episode of depression early in life are at risk for future episodes. Some studies have found that as many as 10 percent of children who have been hospitalized for a suicide attempt will make a successful attempt within the next five years.

The use of antidepressants in children and adolescents is not without controversy, however, according to Theodore Petti, M.D., child and adolescent psychiatrist at Indiana University. While double-blind placebo-controlled studies of hospitalized children have not found much difference in effectiveness between tricyclic antidepressants and placebos, psychiatrists in actual practice *have* found that tricyclics can help ease a child's depression.

The tricyclics are generally the first-choice antidepressants for youngsters because doctors have so much long-term experience with them. "If I see a youngster for a couple of sessions and he doesn't appear to be responding to psychotherapy and he's really hampered in ordinary developmental tasks (such as schoolwork or family relationships), then I will seriously consider using an antidepressant," said Dr. Petti.

While the new SSRIs carry less risk of side effects, there have been no controlled studies among this age group. The major concern that doctors have with using tricyclics in children is the risk of death, presumably from heart problems, that has been associated with the tricyclic desipramine among hyperactive youngsters.

Depression in Adolescence

The picture of depression changes as the child enters adolescence. Many people experience their first bout with major depression during adolescence, although they may not know it. It commonly appears for the first time between ages 15 and 19; recent surveys reveal that as many as 20 percent of high-school students are deeply unhappy or have some kind of psychiatric problem. Suicide is a particular danger for this age group (see box on page 40, "Risk Factors for Teenage Suicide").

Depressed teenagers nearly always experience changes in thinking, such as low self-esteem and self-criticism. In this age group, depression is often disguised as substance abuse. It may be acted out in risk-taking or problems with authority. Depressed teenagers may become antisocial, restless, negative, oversensitive, uncooperative, or aggressive; they may abuse drugs or alcohol and stop going to school. Because most of these symptoms are to some degree considered typical of adolescent behavior in our culture, teenage depression often goes undiagnosed and untreated. This was what happened to Beth.

An 18-year-old athlete who had battled depression and weight problems for most of her teenage years, Beth always blamed her depression on her excess weight, but after shedding 75 pounds, she still felt smothered by a cloak of sadness. She became so despondent that her weight loss had not made her happy that she was driven to hang herself in a tree near her home.

"Even after she lost all that weight," one of her friends recalled, "she smiled with her mouth, but never with her eyes."

Should a teenager you know be thinking of suicide, try to talk about these feelings immediately. Bringing up the subject won't plant ideas that weren't there, but it may help lessen feelings of isolation and entrapment. Ignoring suicidal thoughts or behavior will make suicide more likely to occur.

RISK FACTORS FOR TEENAGE SUICIDE

➤ Previous attempts: Youths who attempt suicide remain vulnerable for several years, especially for the first three months following an attempt.

➤ Psychiatric history: Studies have shown that inpatient psychiatric care is associated with far more suicide attempts.

➤ Personal failure: High standards (the teen's or the parents') that are not met, even after only one setback, may set off a downward spiral ending in suicide.

➤ Recent loss: Death of close friends or family, divorce, or a breakup with a boyfriend or girlfriend may leave a teenager so lost and alone that suicide seems the only option.

➤ Substance abuse: Some teens abuse drugs or alcohol to self-medicate overwhelming depression; a combination of depression, substance abuse, and lowered impulse control can end in a suicide attempt.

➤ Family handguns: A gun in the house may make it easy for a troubled teen to commit suicide; children of law-enforcement officers have a much higher rate of suicide because of the accessibility of guns.

➤ Family violence: Violence in the home teaches youths that the way to resolve conflict is through violence.

➤ Communication lack: The inability to discuss angry or uncomfortable feelings within the family can lead to suicide.

Depression in the Elderly

While older people also suffer from major depression, their condition is often misinterpreted or ignored. Experts estimate that up to 20 percent of the more than 30 million people over age 65 in this country may be experiencing a major depression. In fact, depression is more than 4 times more common in this age group than in the general population, and the suicide rate for people over 65 is 15 times higher.

Depression is *not* a normal part of aging, although it's widely assumed to be, since old age in this country is so often associated with deprivation and loss. In fact, older people are no more "entitled" to feelings of misery than the rest of us.

Because depression in the later years can cause distractibility, indifference, memory problems, and disorientation, the condition is often misdiagnosed as senility. About 12 percent of elderly people who are diagnosed with dementia are really depressed. (It's also possible to be both demented *and* depressed.)

Moreover, many of the diseases that elderly people tend to get may appear as depression. These include Cushing's or Parkinson's disease, thyroid diseases, pulmonary disorders, vitamin deficiencies, cancer, and stroke. Inappropriate sedating drug treatment in nursing-home populations can also cause depression.

If you've been having some personality or mood changes, a doctor should give you a range of tests, including a CAT scan of the brain, blood tests (including thyroid-function tests), and perhaps an electroencephalogram. If these tests don't identify an underlying medical cause for your mood changes, there's a good chance you may be depressed. If you or members of your family have ever been depressed before, this diagnosis is even more likely.

Because metabolism slows with age, elderly people often respond to smaller doses of antidepressants than do younger people.

Treating Depression

As many as 90 percent of people with depression can be successfully treated, usually within 12 to 14 weeks.

One of the first tasks is to choose a mental health professional to diagnose and treat your depression—this could be a psychiatrist, nurse-psychotherapist, social worker, or family therapist. Some people choose a psychotherapist to assist them in understanding and dealing with their problems, and have a psychiatrist or general practitioner prescribe antidepressants and monitor their medical progress.

A psychiatrist has medical training and can prescribe drugs; other mental health professionals have psychotherapy training but can't prescribe medications. In many states, a nurse-psychotherapist may be licensed to prescribe medications in collaboration with a physician.

Of course, what's most important in whomever you choose is that you have trust and confidence in your therapist.

Psychotherapy

Many studies have suggested that the best results can be obtained from a combination of antidepressants and some type of psychotherapy. Even though depression is so responsive to a wide number of drugs, that doesn't mean it's not important to sit down and talk with your doctor to see what the depression is all about.

Talk therapy is probably most useful if your personality and life experiences are the primary cause of your depression. There are a number of different approaches.

Cognitive therapy is based on the idea that depression is a distortion in thinking, that how you feel is a direct product of how you think. Developed specifically to treat depression and anxiety by psychiatrist Aaron T. Beck, M.D., at the University of Pennsylvania, this type of therapy can pinpoint problem patterns of thinking that can result in depressive attitudes.

You'd be surprised how many people—without ever realizing what they're doing—develop a negative pattern of thinking that can automatically lead to depressed feelings. This negative personal outlook can become such a habit that it begins to interfere with everyday functioning.

If you have this problem, you may think that you've caused something to happen that in fact you're not responsible for ("personalization"), or you may exhibit an "all-or-nothing" attitude—believing that unless you're perfect, you've failed. Another typical distortion is "magnification" or "minimization," in which you blow up the importance of some things and discount the value of others.

If you see yourself in this pattern, cognitive therapy can help you understand more about your thought patterns and how to substitute positive thinking. You'll learn how to recognize and label these distortions and understand when you're using them.

Behavioral therapy is similar to cognitive therapy in that it teaches clients how to alter thought distortions, but it also seeks to alter behavior. Based on the idea that a depressed person isn't getting enough positive feedback, this type of therapy offers practical suggestions on how to reinforce healthy behavior via a system of self-rewards. This type of therapy is especially helpful if you have phobias or panic attacks.

Interpersonal therapy focuses on the development and improvement of relationships. Developed by psychiatrist Gerald Klerman, M.D., of Harvard University, and psychologist Myrna Weissman, Ph.D., of Yale University, this type of therapy helps people identify and resolve their problems with others. The client is helped to understand how important positive relationships are to mental health, to assess and define current relationships, and to develop treatment goals. The client is taught relationship skills, focusing on the present instead of the past. Normally considered to be a short-term approach, it doesn't work for everyone. But for appropriate cases, it can be very effective; a 1989 study by the National Institute of Mental Health found that 57 to 69 percent of clients who completed a 16-week course of interpersonal therapy no longer reported depressive symptoms and were more effective at work and at home.

Psychodynamic therapy, much like classical psychoanalysis, explores the past for the seeds of unresolved emotional conflict with a therapist who actively directs the therapy and offers suggestions and interpretations.

You may also benefit from *group therapy*, learning with other people about how best to cope with your depression. Groups can provide a source of connection that helps depressed people interact with others, build new relationships, and benefit from the feedback of others who have been in the same situation. Twelve-step self-help groups can be very effective, since many people are depressed in part because of unresolved addictions. Because an addiction may interfere with depression recovery, participation in such self-help groups may help resolve depression.

But psychotherapy and antidepressants aren't the only ways to deal with depression.

Exercise

There's now solid evidence that regular aerobic exercise (such as running, biking, or swimming) can ease some more moderate cases of depression by raising the level of certain brain chemicals responsible for mood—some of the same brain chemicals that are affected by antidepressants. Even a brisk midday walk for 10 to 20 minutes can help. To be most effective, you should exercise regularly at least three times a week (five times or more is better) for at least half an hour each time.

Don't expect to set Olympic records when you start out, however, or you'll be bound to get discouraged and quit. A combination of walking and running is a good way to start, since it's cheap (no equipment necessary) and you can do it either alone or in a group.

Exercise has not been shown to be effective for severe depression.

Electroshock Treatment

Despite its frightening reputation, electroconvulsive treatment (ECT), formerly known as shock therapy, may work for those very serious depressions that just don't respond to any other treatment, especially when there's a risk of suicide. The modern version of ECT is nothing like the sort of mental torture depicted in movies like *One Flew Over the Cuckoo's Nest*.

While many people believe that the origins of ECT lie in the ancient Roman tradition of applying electric eels to the head as a cure for madness, the true beginning of ECT occurred during the late 1700s. A machine using weak electrical currents was used in Middlesex Hospital in England in 1767 to treat a range of illnesses; London brain surgeon John Birch used this machine to shock the brain of depressed patients. At about the same time, Benjamin Franklin was shocked into unconsciousness (and experienced brief memory loss) during one of his electricity experiments. He is said to have recommended electric shock for the treatment of mental illness.

The modern practice of electric shock treatment for the alleviation of depression and mental illness is less than 65 years old. It was a Hungarian psychiatrist who noticed a number of studies reporting that schizophrenia and epilepsy didn't occur in the same patient; he wondered if an artificially induced seizure might cure schizophrenia.

He began inducing seizures with camphor and other drugs, but Italian psychiatrist Ugo Cerletti and his colleagues explored the possibility of using electric shock to achieve similar results. Cerletti's version was considered an improvement over the drug-induced seizures, which were associated with toxic side effects.

Because it was cheap and easy, the use of ECT soon spread; by the 1950s it was the primary method of treatment for depression until the discovery of antidepressants led to a substantial decline in its use. Today, about 100,000 people in the United States are treated with ECT each year.

How ECT Works. In modern ECT treatments, the patient is given an anesthetic and a muscle relaxant before padded electrodes are applied to one or both of the temples. A controlled electric pulse is delivered to the electrodes until the patient experiences a brain seizure; treatment usually consists of 6 to 12 seizures (two or three a week).

After the treatment, the patient may experience a period of confusion which is later forgotten, and a brief period of amnesia covering the period of time right before the treatment.

On regaining consciousness, patients who have received ECT seem much like those who have experienced post-traumatic amnesia. Tests on memory have revealed a temporary memory impairment; after a number of treatments some patients say they experience a more serious memory loss involving everyday forgetfulness, which usually disappears a few weeks after treatment. New research suggests that ECT given on only one side of the head produces equal benefit to the standard method without any accompanying memory loss.

The controversy surrounding ECT is likely to continue for some time, and it remains unclear whether ECT affects permanent memory. Many studies indicate that ECT doesn't have any extensive effect on permanent memory function. All patients show some amount of amnesia for events immediately before the treatment.

Some scientists believe that some people may falsely conclude that their memory is impaired. In one study, scientists found significant differences between patients who report memory problems and those who don't. Those who complained tended to believe the ECT hadn't helped their depression, which could mean that their own assessment of memory might be the result of their continuing illness. Three years after treatment, this group insisted their amnesia remained, even though there was no objective proof of this. Researchers believe that their initial experience of true amnesia immediately after ECT might have caused them to question whether their memory function had ever recovered.

It is true, however, that ECT in older depressed people who are also demented can worsen their condition. It is also true that ECT can be abused as a treatment. Even ECT proponents admit there is a low incidence of adverse reaction to the treatment, although estimates of how great a risk vary.

ECT in Youth. While depressed teenagers are very much like depressed adults, psychiatrists rarely consider ECT for them, and there are no controlled studies for this age group. In a recent survey, 42 percent of child psychiatrists opposed ECT for young children and 19 percent opposed it for teenagers—even for adolescents with psychotic depression. On the other hand, 100 percent were willing to prescribe antidepressants.

The current attitude against ECT is based on a 1954 study of young schizophrenia patients treated with ECT seven years earlier, which found that benefits were temporary. Since then, more than 100 cases have been published in which results were said to be excellent. For example, a recent Mayo Clinic study of 20 teenagers found that ECT reduced or eliminated symptoms in those with manic-depression and major depression. No adverse effects were reported.

While current research suggests that ECT doesn't harm intellectual development of children or adolescents, there is a risk of prolonged seizure, since youngsters have a greater susceptibility to seizures than do adults. However, according to Max Fink, M.D., professor of psychiatry and neurology at SUNY/Stony Brook, prolonged seizures can be prevented by using less electrical energy, monitoring the duration of the seizure, and cutting the seizure short with an IV of anticonvulsant drugs, such as Valium.

According to Dr. Fink, teenage patients with severe depression or mania who don't respond to medication are often successfully treated with ECT. Too often, however, they are almost always given complex drug combinations that Dr. Fink believes may be more dangerous than ECT and not very effective. He believes that adolescents should be considered candidates for ECT in any situation where it would be appropriate for an adult.

Prepubescent children, however, are another matter. Because of the fear that repeated seizures might damage a maturing brain or interfere with development, it is not often considered to be a good treatment choice. ECT may be used successfully with a few such children suffering from overwhelming impulses to mutilate themselves and who have severe mental retardation.

Is ECT for You? ECT is a rapid, safe, effective treatment for depression. If at least two or three antidepressants have failed to work for you, this may be a good option. An evaluation by a psychiatrist who is very familiar with ECT would be worthwhile if your depression is serious.

Conclusion

This chapter has presented a general overview of depression—what causes it, who's at risk, symptoms, and types of treatment. The next chapter will look at one specific type of treatment—antidepressants. You'll learn how these drugs were developed, their basic biochemical action, and how they might work for you.

2 ALL ABOUT ANTIDEPRESSANTS

"When I was depressed, I was always overwhelmed. It took me so long to do any normal job, just brushing my teeth took forever. I felt doomed all the time. After I took Effexor, I felt as if this terrible weight, this slowing down, had been lifted."

—*Barbara, 49*

There's no *best* way to treat all types of people and depression. In fact, more and more psychiatrists are coming to the conclusion that major recurrent depression is a chronic disease that may require lifetime medication. And while studies suggest that a combination of psychotherapy and antidepressants is the most effective treatment for depression, for some chronically depressed people talk therapy just doesn't help—and it can foster deep feelings of resentment.

"I spent years in group therapy," says Jan, a 39-year-old Boston nurse. "I spent decades talking to experts. I came to realize that I'd put all the honesty a person could muster into my therapy, and I still wasn't any better. Something always felt *physically* wrong. I always felt I had a biochemical twist in me that had to be responsible. If I could only tell the hours, years, the *money* I poured into getting well!"

Finally, a psychiatrist at McLean Hospital in Belmont, Massachusetts, diagnosed Jan as depressed and recommended antidepressants. "Everyone needs a friend," Jan says, "but I think that's where psychotherapy ends—at least for severe depression."

Today there are more than 20 antidepressants on the market, many with fewer side effects than those prescribed a decade ago. Some experts are worried that people will see antidepressants as a quick fix for profoundly complex problems without trying to correct these underlying problems through psychotherapy. Others insist that the drugs simply restore a person's emotional equilibrium, allowing problems to be ironed out without the burden of crushing sadness.

In fact, studies show that combining antidepressants with therapy provides the best chance of treating depression.

Iproniazid: The First Antidepressant

The first of the modern antidepressants—iproniazid—was developed in the early 1950s not to treat depression but to ease the symptoms of tuberculosis. At the time, iproniazid was unmatched as a weapon in the ongoing fight against this deadly respiratory illness, decreasing the number of tubercule bacilli and suppressing their proliferation. But while it was designed to treat tuberculosis, as a side benefit iproniazid also seemed to be a sort of "happy drug," pepping up patients, improving their appetites, and restoring their feelings of well-being.

The drug's positive emotional effects immediately attracted the attention of physicians and depression researchers. The only chemical treatment for depression at that time was opium, a highly addictive substance. The possibility of a more effective—and nonaddictive—drug that could alleviate mood disorders was an attractive thought. Up to that time, some drugs could alleviate one or two symptoms of depression, but none could completely eradicate the condition.

Psychiatrists began to consider using iproniazid as a potential antidepressant just when its manufacturers were getting ready to stop production in the wake of newer, even better-acting antitubercular drugs. With the publication of research in 1957 illustrating the success of iproniazid in the treatment of depression, a flurry of prescriptions were written almost immediately. Within that year, physicians had prescribed it for more than 400,000 depressed patients.

Unfortunately, 127 of them developed jaundice. Although historians believe the jaundice was related to viral hepatitis that was epidemic at that time and not to the iproniazid, its manufacturer withdrew the drug because of adverse publicity.

At about the same time, psychiatrist Roland Kuhn began experimenting with imipramine (Tofranil), the first of the cyclic antidepressants. Imipramine was released in 1958, and amitriptyline (Elavil, Endep, and Amitid) was released soon afterward. Eventually, six other tricyclics were introduced in this country.

After reviewing more than 400 clinical studies of antidepressants, a federal panel of researchers concluded that no one antidepressant was clearly more effective than another, and no one drug successfully treated all cases of depression. Only about half the people find relief with the first antidepressant they are prescribed. This panel also found that psychotherapy together with antidepressants is slightly more effective, helping people understand their problems and relieving stress that may worsen symptoms.

How Antidepressants Work

Although scientists don't know for sure, antidepressants appear to correct a chemical imbalance or dysfunction in the brains of depressed people. An antidepressant boosts the level of neurotransmitters important in fighting depression. Each of the major classes of antidepressants— monoamine oxidase inhibitors (MAOIs), tricyclics, and serotonin inhibitors—affects different neurotransmitter systems in a different way.

Tricyclic antidepressants are a class of traditional drugs that treat depression by boosting the level of several different neurotransmitters (norepinephrine, epinephrine, serotonin, and dopamine) by blocking their reabsorption. MAOIs destroy enzymes responsible for burning up neurotransmitters, thereby boosting the neurotransmitter levels. In general, MAOIs are used to treat those who don't respond to tricyclics. Some of the newest anti-depressants (including Prozac) interfere with the reabsorption of one specific neurotransmitter (serotonin).

Choosing an Antidepressant

Because it seems as if everyone is talking about Prozac, you may be surprised if your doctor doesn't prescribe it right away for your depression. Actually, many doctors feel more comfortable with one of the older antidepressants (tricyclics or MAOIs) because for more than 35 years they've had success prescribing these drugs.

While these drugs do have more side effects than Prozac and other new drugs, many patients can tolerate these problems. More cautious, conservative physicians may choose an "old reliable" despite miraculous claims for the new medications because of worries about unknown long-term effects. If your doctor gives you one of these older drugs and you can't tolerate the side effects or it doesn't help your depression, then he or she may feel more justified in trying one of the newer drugs.

The complex array of brain chemicals and processes that influence depression tends to differ from one patient to the next; because there's no foolproof way to identify what's causing your depression, prescribing antidepressants may be a trial-and-error process until the right one is found.

"My psychiatrist started me out on Zoloft," recalls Linda, 38. "After six weeks, it had done nothing for me, so he switched me to Wellbutrin. I took that for two weeks, but I became oversensitive. So then I was on Prozac for three days, but it made me manic. Then he tried Paxil and added lithium to keep me from getting manic. That's what I've been on for over a year, and it's been great."

Linda's case illustrates the fact that for many people, the first antidepressant is often not the *right* antidepressant. In fact, only a little more than half of all patients who are given antidepressants find relief with their first prescription. No one is quite sure how or why antidepressants work, and no one can predict who will respond to which drug.

"It's a crapshoot," says Dr. Myerson. "We don't have good guidelines about which person will do well on which drug. So we just have to wade through, try different drugs, adjust dosages, and add drugs to drugs. You can have two patients who look identical, but one will respond well to Zoloft and one to Prozac. And we have no idea why."

The best a physician can do is to look at a person's symptoms and try to match those symptoms with an antidepressant. Too often, physicians don't fully explain the side effects and problems a patient may encounter. It's vital to understand the benefits and risks of each antidepressant as you and your physician search for the best treatment.

"Many of my patients don't like to confess that [despite psychotherapy] they are still depressed," one psychiatrist noted. "They feel as if they're letting me down somehow."

There is no one miracle antidepressant that works better than any other, all the time, for everybody. Because depression itself is a complex disease with many causes, doctors must choose from a wide range of antidepressants that work on different brain systems and affect different processes.

When your doctor prescribes an antidepressant, be sure you understand:

> ➤ Which drugs might interact with your antidepressant or cause a toxic reaction.

> ➤ What do you do if you miss one dose—or several doses.

➤ What is the best time of day to take your medication, and how should you take it (on an empty stomach? with food?).

➤ What side effects should you expect and how should you manage them.

➤ How long it will take for the drug to work and how you will know when it's working.

➤ Which side effects are serious enough that you need to contact the doctor immediately.

Combining Drugs

If the first drug fails and your physician has determined that the drug was taken in the right dosage for the correct length of time, he or she may try a different drug. If this second drug also fails, your physician may try combining several different drugs.

When Sara first sought help for her depression, her doctor prescribed an antidepressant and referred her to group therapy. But the first antidepressant didn't seem to do much good—it made her jittery and worsened her sleep problems. When a dosage adjustment didn't improve her symptoms, her psychiatrist switched her to another drug. Sara tried three drugs before finally responding to Zoloft and desipramine, which alleviated her crushing sadness within a few weeks without any other side effects.

Recently, a few psychiatrists—like Sara's doctor—have found that adding desipramine to one of the newer SSRIs such as Prozac or Zoloft seems to work quite well. The dose of each drug is less than would normally be required, so side effects are minimized. A few other drugs, such as thyroid hormone, lithium buspirone (BuSpar), or Ritalin are sometimes added to an antidepressant to boost the drug's effectiveness. While the use of stimulants such as Dexedrine or Ritalin is controversial because of the risk of abuse, adding these drugs to an antidepressant has been successful in alleviating some patients' depression.

If you become psychotically depressed with hallucinations or delusions, your doctor may need to add antipsychotic drugs such as haloperidol (Haldol), risperidone (Risperdal), olanzapine (Zyprexa), or quetiapine (Seroquel) to your antidepressant. Electroconvulsive therapy (ECT) may also be helpful.

Drug combinations can be risky, though, since the more drugs that are given at once, the greater the chance of side effects and drug interactions (such as the dangerous combination of stimulants with MAOIs or certain cyclic antidepressants).

How Long Should You Take Antidepressants?

Length of treatment is becoming controversial. While many people take antidepressants for at least six months to a year, more and more doctors have been suggesting that recurrent depression may be chronic. If you've had more than two episodes of depression, some doctors believe you'll probably need to be on antidepressants for the rest of your life.

On the other hand, it's important not to stop taking antidepressants *too soon*. Research shows that 70 percent of patients become depressed again if they stop taking their antidepressants too early—five weeks or less beyond the point when their symptoms stop. The relapse rate falls to only 14 percent among those who keep taking their antidepressant at least five months after their symptoms abated. Other studies have also found that the longer the patient is on the antidepressant, the less likely is the chance of getting depressed again.

For this reason, many doctors prescribe antidepressants for six months to a year following the end of a depressive episode, gradually tapering off the dosage over several weeks. Unlike opiates, antidepressants aren't addictive, and people taking them will not develop a craving once they are stopped. However, physicians recommend patients gradually taper off the medication to avoid restlessness, anxiety, and other unpleasant physical feelings. This also allows for an opportunity to carefully assess the patient's current need for antidepressant medication.

Side Effects

Side effects from antidepressants generally fall into three categories: sedation; dry mouth, blurry vision, constipation, urinary problems, increased heart rate, and memory problems; and dizziness on standing up (orthostatic hypotension). Drugs that block norepinephrine uptake can produce rapid heartbeat, tremor, and sexual problems. Those that interfere with dopamine (such as Effexor and Asendin) may produce movement disorders and endocrine system changes. Blocking serotonin may create stomach problems, insomnia, and anxiety.

Those that work on the other side of the synapse, blocking receptors that pick up neurotransmitters, have other side effects depending on which receptors are affected. Blocking histamine H_1 receptors produces weight gain and sedation; muscarinic receptor blocks cause dry mouth, constipation, blurry vision, and memory problems.

This is why a tricyclic such as amitriptyline (Elavil) causes so many side effects—it blocks the absorption of both norepinephrine and serotonin, plus four different receptors (alpha$_1$, Dopamine D_2, histamine H_1, and muscarine).

Each drug has a profile of its own particular side effects. Tricyclics often cause dry mouth, constipation, sedation, nervousness, weight gain, and diminished sex drive. MAOIs interact with certain foods and other medications to produce potentially fatal high blood pressure. Newer antidepressants like the SSRIs (such as Prozac, Celexa, Luvox, Paxil, and Zoloft) produce fewer side effects than MAOIs or tricyclics because they affect fewer brain pathways, but nausea and headache may occur.

Although a drug is characterized by certain side effects, that doesn't mean you'll necessarily experience any of them; if you do have persistent side effects, you can switch to a drug with a different side-effect profile. Usually, side effects will disappear or diminish in a week or two. In addition, many antidepressants can be taken before bed so the side effects will occur while you sleep. If a bedtime dose makes you too sleepy the next morning, a dose at dinnertime may be a better idea. A physician can work with your schedule to find the dosage timetable that works best for you.

Many antidepressants lower sex drive; they might cause impotence or interfere in achieving orgasm. These side effects can be eliminated by adding another drug or changing the antidepressant. In most cases, where depression has decreased libido, antidepressants will restore it.

Conclusion

You've just been given a general overview of antidepressants—what they are and how they can help. This book will cover each class of antidepressant, comparing and contrasting them with SSRIs and explaining the details of each one.

In the next chapter, you'll learn about the selective serotonin reuptake inhibitors (SSRIs) like Prozac, the newest class of antidepressants.

3

SELECTIVE SEROTONIN REUPTAKE INHIBITORS (SSRIs)

*"I realized after taking Prozac that I'd been depressed
all my life. I could never really answer the question
'Why do people live? What's the point?' When I was
depressed, I couldn't function. A big day was getting
the newspaper out of the driveway. Now I'm totally
optimistic about everything."*

—Joan, 42, business owner

I t looks ordinary enough, this little green-and-white capsule called Prozac. Not even its manufacturer, Eli Lilly,
claims to know exactly why its product works. But more
than 10 million people have taken this drug for depression,
and more than 70 percent of them have gotten better.
Prozac today is the most popular antidepressant ever.

"I used to walk around with a black cloud over my
head," explains Marie, 41. "I was chronically depressed.
That's how I felt about life; it was an abyss. But after taking
Prozac, my depression is simply gone. I'm not a *different*
person, but I'm a *better* person."

If you've had a depressive episode recently, odds are that the first drug your doctor tries will be one of the SSRIs: Prozac (fluoxetine), Celexa (citalopram), Luvox (fluvoxamine), Zoloft (sertraline), or Paxil (paroxetine).

These drugs have moved to the forefront of modern psychiatric treatment because they work as well as any of the older antidepressants while causing far less serious side effects. Many SSRIs also treat a wide range of other disorders in addition to depression, including obsessive-compulsive disorder (OCD), social phobia, anxiety or panic disorders, post-traumatic stress disorder, eating disorders, premenstrual syndrome (PMS), or menopause-related symptoms.

How SSRIs Work

Remember that the physiological cause of depression lies in the nerve cells in the brain. When the levels of the brain messengers called neurotransmitters are too low, messages can't cross the gaps between brain cells, and communication in the brain slows down. While there are about 100 different kinds of neurotransmitters, the most important ones that seem to be related to depression are serotonin, norepinephrine, and dopamine. When levels of these chemicals are too low, you get depressed. Drugs that boost these chemical levels can relieve depression.

SSRIs target the neurochemical serotonin. When serotonin is released in the brain, it is reabsorbed by the brain cells to be used at another time for another message. This process of reabsorbing is called *reuptake*. If you're depressed, you don't have enough serotonin and other neurotransmitters, so by interfering with the reuptake of these chemicals, more is available to help send messages and boost communication. A drug that can interfere (inhibit) the reabsorption (reuptake) of serotonin alone is "selective"—hence, the selective serotonin reuptake inhibitors.

What makes the SSRIs so attractive is that the older antidepressants tend to affect many different neuro-chemicals and processes in the brain—and the more systems that are altered in the brain, the higher the chance of unpleasant side effects. SSRIs, however, are highly selective, targeting only the problem neurochemical while leaving other brain systems alone.

If you lived in a brand-new custom home and a lightbulb burned out on the second-floor landing, you wouldn't call in an electrician to rip out all the wiring in the walls—you'd just replace the bulb. There's just no need to disrupt all the activities in the entire house to fix one simple problem on the second floor.

It's the same way with depression. If you've got a malfunction in one neurotransmitter system, there's really no need to take a drug that will interfere with other neurotransmitter systems and receptor sites throughout your brain. But for many years, antidepressant drugs did just that.

No one knew how to design a drug that would home in on the lightbulb and ignore the wiring in the rest of the house. Yet it appears that some people do seem to get depressed as a result of something as specific as a malfunctioning serotonin system—the neurological equivalent of a burned-out lightbulb.

For 10 years, scientists searched for this specific drug, looking at different models of nerve transmission and tailoring chemicals to affect these basic processes. They finally found what they'd been looking for in Prozac. With this chemical, scientists finally had a way to simply replace a burned-out bulb without rewiring the whole house.

The beauty of this new class of drugs is that they're so specific. Unlike the shotgun approach of older drugs like tricyclics (see chapter 5) or monoamine oxidase inhibitors (see chapter 6), which interfere with neurotransmitters and receptor sites all over the brain, the SSRIs zero in on serotonin without affecting other brain systems.

The blocking of different neurotransmitters causes different side effects; the greater the number of blocked neurotransmitters, the greater the variety of side effects. For example, blocking the reuptake of norepinephrine can produce tremors, sexual dysfunction, and rapid heart rate. Blocking the reuptake of dopamine can produce movement disorders and changes in the endocrine system. By specifically blocking serotonin alone, you can sidestep most of those problems.

In addition, many of the antidepressants also block receptors on the other side of the synaptic gap that normally absorb the neurotransmitters. Blocking one type of receptor causes sedation and weight gain; blocking another type causes blurred vision, dry mouth, constipation, and memory problems.

It now appears that the serotonin neurotransmitter system may be far more complex than anyone had realized, linking areas throughout the brain in an interwoven tapestry of serotonin-producing connections. Not surprisingly, serotonin receptors are especially plentiful in the areas of the brain controlling emotion. What's more, within the past decade, scientists have realized there are at least six different receptor types in the serotonin system, each responsible for sending different signals to different parts of the brain. The next step is to find a drug that can affect just one of these receptor types, and to develop a simple lab test that can identify specific serotonin malfunctions.

While it's apparent that serotonin is of vital importance in the development of depression, scientists aren't so sure that it's a simple cause-and-effect relationship; the brain's biochemical pathways for emotion and mood are just too complex. While it *may* be true that you can directly relieve depression by increasing serotonin, it could be that monkeying around with serotonin causes slight effects in other neurotransmitter systems, and *those* changes relieve depression.

Prozac: The First SSRI

As the first of the SSRIs to hit the market, by the spring of 1990, Prozac had made the covers of the *New Yorker* and *Newsweek* magazines, touted as the "new wonder drug for depression."

But its early media designation as some sort of happy pill that *every* American might someday want to take to become "better than well" began to raise concerns. Did this drug change behavior, or did it alter personality? It's a sort of chicken-and-egg question that continues to baffle mental health experts. If your mood improves, the outward appearance of your personality and behavior will also change. It stands to reason that if you've been depressed for a long time, you won't have any energy, you might feel negative, you'll mope around, and you might have low self-esteem.

If you take Prozac and your depression improves, you begin to feel more positive, and this makes you feel more self-confident. You may begin to take better care of your appearance. It may *seem* that your entire personality changes. But does it? Where does a mood disorder end and personality begin?

It's important to note that SSRIs like Prozac won't make healthy people "high" the way marijuana or cocaine might. It won't improve your mood if you're already happy, and if you weren't clinically depressed when you took the pill, odds are they won't do a thing for you.

"I was resistant to seeing Prozac as a cure-all," says Miriam, 26, a Virginia artist. "I never felt it was a lifesaver, but it really did give me a calming effect. It got me out of the house, brought me up from the depths, and removed my feeling of panic."

Miriam said she hated her job as salesclerk and, in a happy relationship for the first time, felt panic as she "waited for it all to fall in. When my emotions reached an overwhelming level, I shuffled from one doctor to another until I saw a psychiatrist, who gave me Prozac."

The idea that prescribing Prozac was a sort of "cosmetic psychopharmacology" was promoted by psychiatrist Peter Kramer, author of the best-selling *Listening to Prozac*. In his book, Kramer expressed concern that this antidepressant alters personality as well as illness in a "substantial minority" of users. Actually, Kramer says he doesn't prescribe Prozac that often and notes that it works for a wide variety of problems in addition to depression. His book was not so much for or against Prozac as it was a philosophical exploration of antidepressants and the human personality.

Prime Candidates

After Prozac became available in 1988, it wasn't long before another group of antidepressants in the same class began to appear on pharmacy shelves: Paxil, Zoloft, and Luvox arrived in the mid-1990s, followed by Celexa in 1998.

"Before taking Zoloft, I had a bad case of the blahs. Everything seemed colorless. But now, sometimes I'll just lie in bed and rub the blanket between my fingers," says Sharon, 38. "It's not sexual, but my sensitivity is heightened. The feel-goodness goes right down into my bones."

Research seems to suggest that you can head off serious full-blown illness by taking an SSRI during the early stages of depression. These drugs work so well that someday soon, doctors may begin recommending early screening for depression, just as they now recommend early screening for breast cancer and high blood pressure.

This doesn't mean that SSRIs are the only worthwhile antidepressant, of course. There is still a place for the older drugs. Researchers note that the SSRIs don't work for 20 to 40 percent of depressed or anxious people who try them—the same failure rate as for the older antidepressants. Many of these people find relief either with the newer, structurally unrelated antidepressants such as Wellbutrin, Effexor, or Desyrel, or the "old standby" tricyclics or MAOIs.

Side Effects

The lack of severe side effects is the main reason why this new class of antidepressant has become so popular with doctors and patients alike. That's not to say, of course, that you won't experience *any* side effects with these drugs.

Like most antidepressants, SSRIs may cause nausea, dizziness, or dry mouth, not to mention a range of sexual problems such as decreased or increased sexual interest, ejaculation or orgasm problems, and impotence. When these drugs were first introduced, the manufacturers reported in clinical studies that these sexual problems were rare and occurred in only a few patients. However, a few years in actual practice after several million patients had taken these drugs, physicians found that the incidence of sexual problems was actually much higher. Because many patients may be reluctant to discuss sexual problems with their doctor or pharmacist, the true incidence of these side effects is not known—but many doctors estimate that as many as 70 percent of people who take SSRIs may experience some type of mild sexual problem. (Many other drugs also cause sexual problems, including trycyclics.) Discuss any kind of change in your sexual interest or performance with your doctor while taking SSRIs.

The main difference among all five SSRIs are the side effects they produce. Paxil seems to produce the most drowsiness, which means it can improve sleep for people with insomnia. Zoloft and Luvox appear to cause more gastrointestinal upset (nausea, stomach irritation, diarrhea). Paxil, Prozac, and Zoloft seem to lessen appetite, whereas

Luvox doesn't affect appetite. Paxil has been linked to more complaints of constipation and dry mouth and seems to trigger more pronounced withdrawal symptoms when medication is stopped. All the SSRIs seem to cause problems with sexual interest or performance.

The specific pattern of side effects differs from one SSRI to another and will be discussed in greater detail as each separate drug is described later in the chapter (see box on pages 72 to 73, "Side Effect Comparisons Between SSRIs").

Unlike older antidepressants and lithium, which can be quite toxic, SSRIs are not very dangerous even in high doses. Faced with suicidal patients, many doctors feel more comfortable prescribing an SSRI, since it's unlikely a person could cause permanent damage by taking too much. (In one case, a patient who supposedly took more than 3,000 milligrams of Prozac did not have lasting physical damage.) Also, unlike older antidepressants, the SSRIs appear to be a good choice if you have heart problems or high blood pressure, since they don't appear to affect cardiovascular function.

The SSRIs are also a pleasant change for people who just don't like taking pills, since the total daily dose can be taken as one capsule or tablet (or a liquid, if it's Prozac), compared with three to six pills usually needed for MAOIs or tricyclics.

Finally, unlike the many older antidepressants that cause significant weight gain, most SSRIs don't cause weight gain in many people and may even cause them to lose a few pounds. This is partly because of the mild nausea people feel during the first few days, but it's also because these drugs affect the serotonin system and

SIDE EFFECT COMPARISONS BETWEEN SSRIs

SYMPTOM	CELEXA	LUVOX	PAXIL	PROZAC	ZOLOFT
Agitation	3%	2%			
Amnesia			2%		
Appetite					
Loss		6%	9%	11%	11%
Increase			4%		3%
Blood pressure					
lowering				3%	
Breathing problems		2%			
Chest pain					3%
Concentration problems			3%		
Confusion			1%		
Constipation		10%	16%		8%
Diarrhea	8%	11%	12%	12%	24%
Dizziness		11%	13%	10%	17%
Drowsiness	18%	22%	24%	13%	15%
Fatigue	5%				14%
Fever	2%			2%	2%
Flulike symptoms		3%		5%	
Gas		4%	4%	3%	4%
Headache		22%	18%	21%	30%
Heart pounding		3%	3%	2%	4%
Indigestion				8%	
Insomnia	15%	21%	24%	20%	28%
Itching				3%	
Mouth dryness	20%	14%	18%	10%	16%
Muscle pain					
Pain			1%		
Numbness			1%		
Tension					2%
Tightness		2%			
Nausea	21%	40%	26%	23%	30%

SIDE EFFECT COMPARISONS BETWEEN SSRIs *(continued)*

SYMPTOM	CELEXA	LUVOX	PAXIL	PROZAC	ZOLOFT
Numbness			4%		3%
Paranoia					2%
Rash			3%	4%	
Sexual problems					
Male			10%		
Female			3%		2%
Ejaculation	6%		23%		17%
Loss of interest	2%	2%	7%	4%	11%
Impotence	3%	2%	8%		5%
Orgasm		2%			
Sweating	11%	7%	11%	8%	8%
Taste change		3%	2%		3%
Throat soreness				5%	4%
Tremors	8%	5%	11%	10%	11%
Twitching					1%
Urination					
Problems			3%		
Increase		3%	3%		2%
Vomiting	4%	5%		3%	4%
Weight					
Increase					3%
Loss				2%	

lessen carbohydrate craving. This benefit shouldn't be downplayed, psychiatrists say, since the weight gain caused by the older antidepressants—which could be 30 pounds or more—could be a real stumbling block to staying on the drug.

This does *not* mean that these drugs are some sort of diet pill. It's more likely to prevent weight gain than to initiate weight loss. Not *everybody* who takes these drugs loses weight, and most only lose a pound or two. Researchers note that the heaviest people are those who tend to lose a few pounds on SSRIs, while the slimmest users are the ones most likely to gain.

Withdrawal

Continued use of SSRIs can lead to a "discontinuation syndrome" after a patient abruptly stops taking the medication. Symptoms may include dizziness, dry mouth, insomnia, nausea, nervousness, and sweating. For this reason, if you have taken an SSRI for more than one week you should taper the dose for another week to minimize the risk of these symptoms. If you've taken the drug for more than six weeks, you should taper the dose gradually over a two-week period.

Other Disadvantages

What concerns some doctors is that the long-term effects of the SSRIs are largely unknown. A series of studies in humans has shown no connection between antidepressant use and cancer, but there are some concerns about whether antidepressants promote tumor growth in cancer patients or those exposed to cancer-causing substances (such as nicotine in cigarettes). This concern is primarily due to a small study published in 1992 that found that after being injected with cancer cells or cancer-causing substances, rats subsequently injected with antidepressants had more tumors than did control rats.

Cost is also an issue. Older antidepressants like the MAOIs and the tricyclics are cheaper than SSRIs because their patents have expired, making them less expensive compared to the newest SSRIs. No matter how wonderful a drug may be, if you can't afford it, it's not going to do you much good. The high cost of the SSRIs can be a real hardship for someone with no insurance, or whose insurance doesn't cover drugs. At about $2 per pill, the pharmacy bill can be overwhelming.

It is a problem for Mary, 28, whose health insurance covers all drugs *except* medications for mental health problems. "My psychiatrist is very aware of this problem," Mary explains. "He doesn't give me Zoloft alone because it would be too expensive. So he prescribes a smaller amount of Zoloft with desipramine [a less expensive tricyclic]." The desipramine boosts the effects of Zoloft, and the combination costs less than a full dose of Zoloft alone.

Tolerance is also a concern. (A person develops drug "tolerance" when the drug suddenly stops working, requiring larger and larger doses to be effective.) About 1 in 50 patients will develop tolerance to any drug, doctors say, and there have been reports of tolerance with SSRIs.

Sherry, 38, has suffered for some time with many health problems, including obesity and chronic pain from arthritis. Depressed over these health worries, she began taking one capsule of Prozac daily, which eased her depression at first. She's now up to five tablets daily (100 milligrams), a very high dose indeed.

"The crying episodes have stopped," she reports, "but Prozac is not just effective anymore. Before I was always able to pull myself back from depression. Now I'm just crazed, and I've lost faith in traditional medicine."

Which SSRI Is Best?

Research suggests that all the SSRIs are about equally effective—but each drug has a certain profile of its own particular side effects. And for some reason, some people respond better to one than to another. No one knows exactly why. So how does your doctor decide which drug to give you? Most physicians have personal "favorites" as a first-option treatment, based on the past experiences of other patients. Beyond that, it's trial and error.

Your doctor may start you out on Zoloft; if you don't respond after three or four weeks, you may be switched to another SSRI, such as Paxil or Prozac. Doctors can keep trying SSRIs (and then begin with the older antidepressants) until you respond.

Effectiveness

While studies suggest that all five SSRIs are equally effective, each person's unique chemical makeup and the level of the disease itself affects how every drug works.

In addition, while all these drugs tend to stay in the body for some time, some remain longer than others. Prozac has the longest half life, which is of concern if you are having unpleasant side effects with this drug. If you've been taking Prozac for a few weeks on a regular basis, it may take up to five weeks before all of the drug and its metabolites are excreted.

Zoloft will remain in the body for at least three to five days, Paxil for at least 42 hours, Luvox for at least 32 hours, and Celexa for at least three days.

All these drugs usually take between two to four weeks before improvement begins. While it is sometimes possible for some patients to experience relief within the first week, most take longer before symptoms ease.

Interactions

All SSRIs have similar interactions with many drugs; the most serious is a possible fatal interaction with the antidepressant class of MAOIs. For this reason, you should allow at least two weeks to pass between stopping one of these drugs and starting one from the other class. With Prozac, you should wait between five to six weeks before taking an MAOI (and two weeks for the reverse).

Of all these drugs, Luvox seems to be the one likely to cause serious problems when taken with other drugs. For specific drug interactions, see each individual drug listing later in this chapter.

Combining Antidepressants

While you may be started out on a single antidepressant, the current trend in treatment-resistant depression is toward combinations of two medications, either to boost their efficiency or to counteract potential side effects. For example, Desyrel (an antidepressant unrelated to SSRIs or older drugs) is sometimes added to Prozac if a patient has trouble sleeping when taking Prozac alone.

"I take Desyrel right before I go to sleep," says Sarah, 42. "Before taking antidepressants, I was having a lot of trouble sleeping because of my depression. But Prozac didn't help that. So after a few weeks on Prozac, my psychiatrist added Desyrel, and I started sleeping again for the first time in years."

Some research suggests that a combination of Prozac and lithium may help some people who don't improve on either drug alone.

SSRIs and Older Patients

All five drugs work well for older people, and experts consider that all are about equally effective. However, research suggests that older patients taking Paxil or Luvox will have much higher blood levels of the drug compared to younger patients. For this reason, some doctors prescribe lower doses of these drugs for older people or monitor their response more closely.

SSRIs and Children

Luvox is the only SSRI of the five currently approved for use in children (and only for obsessive-compulsive disorder). However, all the SSRIs have been prescribed for thousands of younger patients as an "off label" use, not just for depression but for obsessive-compulsive disorder, anxiety, panic, and ADHD. Since depression can appear in children at least as young as six (and often younger), the ability to treat childhood depression is important. Depression is one of the most common mental illnesses in children, affecting about 2 percent of all youngsters in the United States.

Unfortunately, there is not much definitive research showing how these drugs affect children—for better or worse. Many experts are concerned about potential long-term effects of these drugs, especially since young children are still passing through a variety of growth and development stages that may be affected by antidepressants.

Most studies of SSRIs in children have been conducted with Luvox as a treatment for OCD. These studies have found that Luvox is not only effective in young patients, but that younger children seem to experience different side effects that aren't noticed in adults, such as abnormal thinking, muscle twitching, or bloody or stuffy nose.

Some doctors prefer starting young patients on different drugs, but in general, most prefer prescribing one of the SSRIs that must be given only once a day (Luvox is dosed twice daily). Prozac is often a first choice because it is available as a liquid, making it much easier to give to children younger than 12 who can't swallow pills easily. In addition, in selecting an SSRI for a child, a doctor may choose the same antidepressant that has worked well for someone else in the child's family.

Pregnant and Breast-feeding Women

All the five SSRIs are classified by the FDA as pregnancy category C, from a list that ranges A (safest) to D (least safe). Antidepressant use should be discussed with your obstetrician.

Because Prozac, Paxil, and Luvox are found in breast milk, you should not take these drugs while breast-feeding. While it isn't known if Zoloft and Celexa are passed through breast milk, most experts believe that you should not breast-feed if you're taking these drugs, either.

SSRIs and Other Disorders

Many antidepressants are prescribed not just to treat depression, but for a wide variety of other conditions related to mental health.

When a drug is first approved by the FDA, the government specifies which conditions the drug has been proven to treat effectively. However, doctors may prescribe the drug for other conditions, even if the FDA has not officially approved the drug for those situations. This is called an "off label" use, and it's perfectly legal. Once a drug company has done additional studies to prove that the drug also works for these new conditions, the company can ask the FDA to officially approve the drug for these new uses.

The FDA has approved the following "new" uses of SSRIs:

> ➤ *OCD:* Zoloft, Prozac, Paxil, and Luvox are approved for the treatment of OCD (Celexa isn't); but only Luvox is approved to treat OCD in children

> ➤ *Bulimia:* Prozac

> ➤ *Generalized anxiety disorder:* Paxil

> ➤ *Geriatric depression:* Prozac

➤ *Mania:* Zyprexa has been approved to treat mania in patients with bipolar disorder (manic-depression)

➤ *Panic disorder:* Paxil and Zoloft

➤ *PMS (severe):* Prozac (marketed as Sarafem)

➤ *Post-traumatic stress disorder (PTSD):* Zoloft and Paxil

➤ *Social anxiety disorder:* Paxil

New studies also have been done suggesting that certain other SSRIs work for conditions not yet approved by the FDA:

➤ *Cognitive performance in the elderly:* all antidepressants

➤ *Menopause symptoms:* all antidepressants

➤ *Hot flashes:* Paxil

➤ *Geriatric depression:* Celexa

➤ *PTSD:* Zoloft

➤ *PMS:* Effexor

The SSRIs have also been used to treat a wide variety of other disorders, including nicotine withdrawal, exhibitionism, Tourette's syndrome, and even itchy skin under certain circumstances. People with body dysmorphic disorder (the false perception that part of the body is abnormal) generally feel better with an SSRI. Several studies have found that Prozac may also help alcoholics decrease the amount of alcohol they drink; while other

SSRIs increased the number of days that alcoholics can abstain from drinking. Studies suggest that Prozac can improve functioning in patients suffering from either schizophrenia or borderline personality disorder. Schizophrenics, for example, may become less aggressive and more interested in social activities.

Prozac

First introduced in 1988, Prozac singlehandedly helped remove the stigma of mental illness, proving to many skeptics that depression is really a disease, not a moral weakness. Once the nation's top-selling antidepressant, demand for the little green capsule has faded since new drugs promising increased effectiveness with fewer side effects have arrived on the market. In January 2000, doctors wrote more prescriptions for Zoloft than for Prozac.

The first of a new generation of drugs, the SSRIs, Prozac had far fewer side effects than traditional antidepressants yet worked surprisingly well not just for depression but for many other mental problems, as well. Since then, about 17 million Americans have taken Prozac, and by 1999, its manufacturer, Eli Lilly, recorded worldwide sales of $2.61 billion.

Criticized in the past for making a few patients more self-destructive or suicidal, the attacks eventually faded as Prozac continued its momentum.

But eventually, Prozac's star was destined to fade, since very few prescription drugs stay at the crest of the market for more than five or six years due to incredible competition from newer drugs and generics. Newer

SSRIs, Celexa, Paxil, and Zoloft, have all launched ad campaigns promising fewer problems with fatigue and waning libido that are more common with Prozac. Experts say there's not much actual difference between Prozac, Zoloft, and Paxil (the three top antidepressants), but for unknown reasons, some patients respond better to one antidepressant than to another.

How Prozac Is Administered

You'll probably be started out on 10 to 20 milligrams daily, and if you haven't responded within a month, your dosage may be increased to as much as 40 milligrams. Most patients don't take more than 80 milligrams, however, and some studies suggest that lower doses usually work better. (In a few cases, very obese people have responded to doses over 80 milligrams, although this excessive dosage is not recommended in general because of safety concerns.)

A once-a-week version of Prozac, Prozac Weekly, was approved in March 2001. Prozac Weekly's manufacturer convinced the FDA that it was as effective as daily Prozac for people who had already been taking the old version of the drug and that side effects were also similar. Available as a 90-milligram pill, Prozac Weekly is expected to be less expensive and easier for patients to take, since they only have to take it once a week.

However, some pharmacology experts suggest that the force behind the drug's development had less to do with treatment than with patent rights. Eli Lilly's exclusive right to sell fluoxetine (the drug's chemical name) expired

August 2001, and the company has been searching for variations that would carry on some patent protection.

Experts don't believe there will be weekly versions of other antidepressants, since Prozac Weekly takes advantage of fluoxetine's uniquely slow metabolization rate.

Like all antidepressants, Prozac doesn't work overnight. It will usually take two to three weeks before you start to notice a difference in how you're feeling, although some people insist their depression improves within the first week. In most cases, depression lifts within one to two months. You should take the full dose for at least six weeks before deciding that it's not going to work. If you do have a good response, most doctors recommend you continue taking Prozac for six to eight months before stopping. If you're contemplating stopping, it's better to wait until you appear to have no upcoming stress, such as divorce proceedings or a major sales presentation. When you and your doctor decide it's time to stop taking Prozac, your doctor will teach you how to tell if your depression is returning.

Withdrawal

Prozac rarely produces withdrawal symptoms when you stop taking it. Because of its long half-life, you can usually stop taking Prozac abruptly without complications. However, some doctors suggest you taper off your doses and closely watch for any indication of a relapse.

If you begin to feel lethargic, have low moods, or experience appetite or sleep problems, your depression could be returning. *These are not the symptoms of any sort of withdrawal.* If it is your depression returning, you can start taking Prozac again and it should work as well as it did before.

Unfortunately, some people do experience depression again and again. Because of the underlying biological component of depression, there's at least a 50 percent chance you may experience another episode. For those who've already had two episodes, the chances of a third jump to about 90 percent. Therefore, for cases of recurrent depression, experts today sometimes recommend taking Prozac indefinitely to prevent future occurrences.

Side Effects

The most frequent complaint about Prozac is nausea; you may not feel very hungry for the first few days. But this nausea usually disappears after about two weeks. It may help to take your medication with a meal, or to divide your dose in half for a while; ask your doctor about this. If your nausea doesn't go away in a week or two, or it gets worse, you may have to switch to another antidepressant.

Other common side effects include nervousness and anxiety. Prozac can be very stimulating, and some people feel a caffeinelike buzz after taking this drug. "When I take Prozac, I feel jittery," Joan says, "sort of like drinking five pots of coffee. Other than that, I don't have any physical side effects."

Prozac's stimulatory properties can also cause sleep problems in some people, probably because Prozac (like other SSRIs) affects serotonin, which is responsible for regulating the sleep-wake cycle. Fortunately, only about 2 percent of patients find the insomnia so troubling that they are forced to stop taking Prozac. About the same percentage are equally disturbed by the drowsiness they experience with this drug. If you do experience insomnia, you can try taking your medicine earlier in the day, or ask your doctor about combining Prozac with Desyrel (trazodone).

About 9 percent of people taking Prozac report dry mouth, compared to about 65 percent of those taking tricyclics. A few people also notice sweating, tremors, or rash.

Most antidepressants (except for Wellbutrin) cause some degree of sexual problems, and Prozac isn't any different. Between 40 and 70 percent of people experience negative sexual side effects, including delayed ejaculation, impotence, decreased libido, or problems reaching orgasm. Patients cite loss of sexual interest as one of the biggest problems with Prozac. On the other hand, some people feel *more* interested in sex than before, possibly because depression had interfered with their libido.

More seriously, Prozac can induce a manic state (excess elation, hyperactivity, agitation, and speeded-up thinking and talking) in people who are inclined to be manic-depressive. This is a real problem, and it's something your doctor will be monitoring, especially if there's a history of manic-depression in your family. Your doctor may want to cut back your dose or combine Prozac with lithium to manage the mania. Some people may have to stop the drug completely.

"Prozac made me speed," says Julie, a 38-year-old with a family history of manic-depression. "I was scouring every nook and cranny. I had two vacuums going in the bedroom at once, one for the corners and one for the floor. I hadn't cleaned that much for two years because I was depressed. Once I took Prozac, suddenly I felt like doing a *really good job*. The night before I went on the cleaning binge, I lay in bed for two hours thinking that I could smell the dust. As soon as I told my psychiatrist, he immediately took me off Prozac and put me on Paxil."

The main difference between Prozac and other SSRIs is that Prozac stays in the body much longer. Up to six weeks after you stop taking the drug, traces of Prozac and its metabolites can still be found in your body. What this means is that if you have a bad reaction to Zoloft or Paxil, the unpleasant symptoms may linger for a week or two. But adverse effects from taking Prozac can last up to six weeks after you've stopped taking the drug.

There's a benefit to this, however. You'll be less likely to experience a relapse of depression if you forget a dose or two of Prozac, and you'll be less likely to have withdrawal effects from suddenly discontinuing the drug.

Drug Interactions

There's nothing wrong with taking both Prozac and over-the-counter pain medications like Tylenol or Advil. And while a few reports suggest that Prozac slows down the rate at which the body breaks down antianxiety drugs, such as Valium (diazepam), this doesn't appear to cause any serious problems. Lots of people who are depressed are also anxious, and many people take Valium as part of their treatment. A slowdown in the metabolism rate of Valium simply means the drug will remain in your body for a slightly longer period.

Prozac mixed with tricyclics or a tetracyclic such as Ludiomil isn't dangerous, although Prozac can enhance the effects of these drugs and cause insomnia, appetite loss, and anxiety. And the risk of heart problems and seizure already associated with tricyclics increases when Prozac is added.

But it's *very* dangerous to take Prozac—or any SSRI—with MAOIs (such as Nardil or Parnate). This combination could cause a fatal reaction, including nausea and vomiting, high blood pressure, and shock. This is why you should wait at least two weeks after taking an MAOI before taking Prozac, and at least five weeks *after* taking Prozac before taking an MAOI.

Food Interactions

Food doesn't affect the blood levels or amount of Prozac absorbed from the stomach; you can take it with either food or beverages (and if the drug makes you feel nauseated, taking it with food or milk may help ease the discomfort).

Suicide

According to a series of very large studies including one published in the *British Medical Journal,* there is no evidence of increased suicide risk or suicidal thoughts among people taking Prozac. In the study, Prozac caused fewer substantial suicidal thoughts than did tricyclics or placebo. Of those people who did have suicidal thoughts when they started taking Prozac, those given a placebo had the highest increase in those thoughts, with Prozac showing the least increase (17.9 percent for placebo, 16.3 percent for tricyclics, and 15.3 percent for Prozac).

If you're depressed, it's possible you might have some suicidal thoughts; between 40 and 60 percent of people with major depression do. Tell your doctor immediately if you start feeling self-destructive.

Prozac and Obsessive-Compulsive Disorder

Since Prozac affects the serotonin system, and because serotonin has been implicated in a host of other disorders, it's not surprising that Prozac appears to help lots of other problems besides depression.

In July 1993, the FDA approved Prozac for the treatment of obsessive-compulsive disorder. This disorder is surprisingly common in this country, affecting 5 million Americans with symptoms commonly beginning as early as age 10.

People with OCD become obsessed with certain thoughts and bogged down with repetitive activities, like washing their hands or rechecking doors and windows. (A "compulsion" is a rigid behavior that is repeated over and over every day.) If you have OCD, you may be fearful about dirt, disease, or toxic chemicals, or you may need to count, align, check, or apologize constantly.

People with OCD are not out of touch with reality. They *know* their behavior isn't reasonable, and about a third are so upset about their problem that they become clinically depressed.

Studies have shown that Prozac can help up to 70 percent of people with OCD, although it can take up to 10 weeks to notice improvement. Patients usually take higher doses of Prozac for OCD on a long-term basis. And because Prozac does not carry many of the harmful side effects that interfere with antidepressant use in children, it has been given to young OCD patients with favorable results. One study reported that four out of eight youngsters given up to 80 milligrams of Prozac daily completely stopped their handwashing rituals after two months.

Luvox (fluvoxamine) and the tricyclic Anafranil (clomipramine) are also very effective treatments.

Prozac and Eating Disorders

Bulimia. Prozac has been approved for the treatment of bulimia, a sometimes-fatal disorder of compulsive eating binges and self-induced vomiting and laxative abuse. Estimates of bulimia sufferers range from 1 to 10 percent of all American women and up to 14 percent of college-age women.

Some research suggests that depression can be an underlying cause of eating disorders; one study of bulimics found that three out of four bulimic patients were depressed.

Studies suggest that Prozac can help ease eating binges in up to 63 percent of people with bulimia nervosa. While MAOIs also help with bulimia, the side effects and rigid diet restrictions often cause problems for patients. And because many patients taking MAOIs gain weight, the chance is small that patients will stick with this medication regimen considering their intolerable fear of weight gain. In fact, a recent study of 27 bulimic patients found that while they responded well to the drug, 24 stopped taking the drug within four months because of the side effects.

Some scientists believe that Prozac may be helpful in correcting bulimia because it reduces appetite; some studies found that rats given fluoxetine and then deprived of their favorite food for a day ate less than they would normally eat. Other experts believe the drug corrects the underlying serotonin malfunction, pointing out that other antidepressants that don't affect appetite but do affect serotonin are also effective against bulimia.

In another study, up to 65 percent of bulimic patients responded to antidepressants, although many did not respond to the first drug that was tried. In this particular study, 6 of the 17 patients who experienced remission of their symptoms were taking Prozac.

A combination of psychotherapy and Prozac has been the most effective treatment for bulimia.

Anorexia Nervosa. Anorexic patients have antidepressant needs that are a little different from bulimic subjects. Still, a new study by the University of Pittsburgh Medical Center found that Prozac can help patients with anorexia. When 16 women with the eating disorder were given Prozac, 10 stayed at a healthy weight and didn't relapse, while only 3 of 19 anorexic women placed on a placebo were able to remain healthy. This study is the first to show an antidepressant could help prevent anorexia relapses, according to study director Walter Kaye, M.D. Prozac may help by altering brain chemicals that affect both mood and appetite. Experts were hopeful because a medication that can help patients maintain a healthy weight outside of a hospital and prevent relapse can ultimately save lives. Currently, there is no anorexia treatment that has been approved by the FDA.

What Prozac and other antidepressants can do is to address the underlying biological problem that may be causing the eating disorder; this treatment, combined with supportive psychotherapy and nutritional counseling, may help break the cycle of anorexia.

Prozac and Premenstrual Syndrome

If you suffer from premenstrual syndrome (PMS), your doctor may well prescribe Prozac, which was approved to treat severe PMS in the year 2000. However, it is marketed under a different name, Sarafem, to catch women's attention. It's the exact same drug as Prozac, but the Sarafem version comes with a brochure explaining PMS—known medically as premenstrual dysphoric disorder, or PMDD. Sarafem comes in seven-day blister packs to help women keep track of their use.

Between 3 and 5 percent of women during child-bearing years experience typically mild PMS each month, with complaints ranging from breast tenderness and bloating to anxiety and mood swings some time between ovulation and menstruation. But some women who suffer extremely strong symptoms, including irritability and depression, actually have PMDD.

In the past, doctors had prescribed Prozac for these women (and also Zoloft and Celexa), although the FDA had not specifically approved them as PMDD treatments. While it is legal for a doctor to prescribe a drug for off label use, FDA approval allows a manufacturer to market a drug for a specific condition.

Sarafem is the only drug indicated for the treatment of PMDD. Studies suggest that women taking the drug had significant improvements in both mood and physical symptoms—improvements which appeared during the very first menstrual period. The prescription-only Sarafem pack is sold at the same price as Prozac and carries the same side effects.

Pregnancy and Breast-feeding

Animal studies haven't found any problems with taking Prozac during pregnancy, even in 11 times the normal human dosage. However, it's rated as pregnancy category C by the FDA.

A study in the January 1997 *New England Journal of Medicine* concluded that taking Prozac during pregnancy doesn't affect the IQ, language development, or behavior of the child, at least throughout the preschool years. In a study of more than 200 preschoolers, there also were no significant differences in temperament, mood, activity level, distractibility, or other problems, according to researchers at the University of Toronto in Ontario, Canada. Moreover, there were no developmental differences between infants who were exposed to antidepressants only during the first three months of pregnancy and those whose mothers took the drugs throughout pregnancy.

Previous research has shown that infants who were exposed to the antidepressants in the womb were no more likely to have major birth defects than those who were never exposed. Although one study indicated that taking Prozac during the third trimester of pregnancy might lower an infant's birth weight and increase the risk of preterm delivery, the new study found no evidence of such problems.

At the time the children were born and when they were tested for learning and behavioral problems, their weights and heights were similar regardless of whether their mothers had taken an antidepressant during pregnancy. Moreover, the study found that women who had taken the drugs during pregnancy were no more likely to give birth prematurely than those who hadn't taken them.

Because depression during pregnancy is a big problem, birthing experts felt reassured that at last there are some reassuring data about the safety of these drugs. Untreated depression can have a negative effect on pregnancy, especially if a woman has problems eating or sleeping.

While this study is encouraging, experts really can't be certain yet about the safety and effects of antidepressant use during pregnancy. Some doctors recommend that, if at all possible, you not use Prozac (or any other antidepressant) if you're pregnant or trying to conceive, but it is usually considered safe today. However, if you become severely depressed without medication during pregnancy, you and your doctor must weigh the severity of the depression with the available information on how the drug might affect a developing fetus.

Like most antidepressants, Prozac is secreted in mother's milk. Since scientists just don't know what effect this might have on the baby, most doctors recommend that you not plan to breast-feed if you're taking Prozac. You'll need to weigh these decisions, however, since Prozac and many other antidepressants *are* effective in treating postpartum depression.

Prozac and Older Patients

If you're over 65 and depressed, chances are you'll respond just as well to Prozac as you would to a number of other antidepressants (such as nortriptyline, a tricyclic). However, because side effects like dry mouth and constipation aren't such a problem with Prozac and the other

SSRIs, you're more likely to be able to tolerate treatment. And Prozac is ideal for older people because it doesn't interfere with blood pressure or heart function. In fact, Prozac and the other SSRIs (plus Wellbutrin) are among the safest antidepressants for people with heart disease.

Prozac is the first antidepressant that has specific FDA approval for use in geriatric depression. The approval comes in the wake of a 1997 FDA ruling that requires all medications to have a "geriatric use" section in their label, with information about safety for older patients.

There have been a few reports noting that some older people taking Prozac have low levels of sodium in their blood, causing them to retain water, which can lead to swelling. Your doctor will advise you if you are likely to experience this problem.

Prozac and Children

Prozac is not currently approved for use in children with depression, although it is often prescribed for them. A few studies suggest that children and adolescents may be given Prozac provided they are carefully screened for manic-depression in themselves or their family.

Prozac doesn't appear to cause the cardiovascular problems in children that sometimes occur with other antidepressants, and it is effective against both bulimia (so troubling in adolescence) and obsessive-compulsive disorder, which often appear in childhood.

Studies suggest that younger people respond with very small doses, possibly as small as 5 to 10 milligrams daily to start. And a sizable portion of young people who do not respond to other antidepressants do respond to Prozac.

Studies also suggest that younger people experience slightly different side effects than those experienced by older patients. Restlessness and sweating are the most commonly reported side effects, together with drowsiness, dry mouth, tremors, and thinning hair.

Cost

Although prices vary from one part of the country to another, you can generally expect to pay between $55 and $100 for 30 capsules of Prozac (10 to 20 milligrams) and between $105 and $160 for 4 ounces of liquid Prozac.

However, that price could soon decrease significantly when Prozac's patent expires and generic versions of Prozac enter the market. Already generic versions are available in Great Britain and other parts of Europe. Despite opposition from Prozac's manufacturer, Eli Lilly, a generic version of Prozac could become available sometime in 2001. However, further appeals could put off a generic version until 2003. To head off potential losses, Prozac manufacturers paid the Massachusetts-based company Sepracor for the right to sell a modified form of Prozac that promises a more effective treatment for depression, with fewer side effects such as sexual dysfunction and impotence and the inner tension that some critics say could lead to violence. (Eli Lilly still denies that Prozac causes violence or suicide in any way.)

When the new version is introduced in 2002, it might allow Eli Lilly to retain its franchise on the nation's most popular antidepressant, even if generic versions hit the market when the drug's main patent expires in 2003. Many doctors may prefer to prescribe the new Prozac, which could be seen as superior to cheaper generic versions of the original Prozac. No generic versions of the new Prozac could be produced until 2015.

Who Should Take Prozac Cautiously

Obviously if you're allergic to Prozac (indicated by hives or a rash), you shouldn't take this antidepressant. And if you have serious problems with your liver or kidneys, it's not a good idea to take Prozac because this drug is metabolized in the liver and excreted in the kidneys. If you have serious problems with either of these organs, Prozac could build up in your blood to toxic levels.

You should also be cautious about taking Prozac if you have a history of seizures or epilepsy, even if you're taking antiseizure medication. Studies of more than 6,000 people revealed that 12 patients experienced seizures with Prozac, about the same rate as that of other antidepressants. If you have such a history, your doctor will want you to have a full neurological workup with an EEG before proceeding. You'll have to take smaller-than-usual doses at first, and you'll probably need a series of EEGs and blood tests (to monitor anticonvulsant levels) during treatment.

Celexa

The newest SSRI is Celexa (citalopram HBr), approved for the treatment of depression by the FDA in the summer of 1998. A highly selective serotonin reuptake inhibitor,

Celexa is the best-selling antidepressant in 13 other countries. Celexa offers help to a broad range of patients, both improving depression and preventing relapse, and was well-tolerated in studies of more than 23,000 people over 10 years. It has helped more than 8 million people in the 64 countries where it has been available.

You should take Celexa once a day in the morning or evening, with or without food. Your doctor will probably begin with a 20-milligram daily dose, increasing it to 40 milligrams if you don't respond. Although certain patients may require a dose of 60 milligrams a day, studies haven't found that this higher dosage is any more effective than is 40 milligrams. Improvement may take between one week and one month.

The risk of fatal overdose using Celexa alone is low; of the 12 reported overdose fatalities, 10 occurred when Celexa was combined with other drugs and/or alcohol. The two fatal cases when Celexa was used alone were at overdoses of 3,920 milligrams and 2,800 milligrams; there were also reports of nonfatal overdoses at up to 6,000 milligrams.

Side Effects

Side effects reported with Celexa were generally mild and tend to fade away during treatment. Frequent (but mild) side effects include nausea, dry mouth, sweating, insomnia, tremor, diarrhea, and sleepiness. As with all SSRIs, Celexa should be used with caution in patients with a history of mania or seizures.

In at least 1 out of 100 patients, other symptoms include low blood pressure, dizziness when standing up, rapid heartbeat, headache, excessive saliva, flatulence, weight loss or gain, poor concentration, amnesia, apathy, increased appetite, confusion, cessation of menstrual periods, coughing, rash, itching, and taste problems. Like most SSRIs, Celexa appears to interfere with many aspects of sexual experience and function, particularly ejaculation delays, decreased sex drive, lack of orgasms, and impotence.

Drug Interactions

One of the strengths of this SSRI is that there are few drug interactions. The manufacturer does not recommend combining alcohol with Celexa, and you should tell your doctor if you take (or plan to take) any prescription or over-the-counter medication. Certain drugs may affect the strength of blood medication levels or slow down clearance from the body, including:

> ➤ *Cimetidine:* This drug raises the blood level of Celexa

> ➤ *Antifungal drugs:* There is a potential that these drugs (ketoconazole, itraconazole, fluconazole, or omeprazole) may slow down the clearance of Celexa from the body

> ➤ *Erythromycin:* This antibiotic may potentially slow down the clearance of Celexa from the body

> ➤ *Tricyclics:* Celexa doubles the concentration of a metabolite of imipramine

> ➤ *MAOIs:* As with all SSRIs, severe potential side effects can occur if taken within two weeks of a MAOI antidepressant

Pregnancy and Breast-feeding

Celexa is classified as pregnancy category C by the FDA due to abnormal effects on animal fetus development and birth when given higher-than-normal human doses, including stillbirth, decreased birth weight, and perinatal death. Based on animal studies, it's important to weigh the risk of damage to the fetus against the risk of going without the antidepressant during pregnancy. Because there were no adequate or well-controlled studies in pregnant women, the manufacturer advises that Celexa should be used during pregnancy only if the potential benefit to the mother justifies the potential risk to the fetus.

Celexa is passed through breast milk and there were two reports of infants experiencing sleepiness, decreased feeding, and weight loss. The manufacturer recommends that treatment should balance the risks of Celexa exposure for the baby and the benefits for the mother.

Celexa and Older Patients

Studies on older patients determined that Celexa was just as safe and effective for younger and older adults, although blood concentrations were higher and the drug stayed in the body longer among older patients. Because Celexa has little potential to affect the metabolism of other drugs, it may be a good choice for senior citizens. Most older people in the Celexa studies received daily doses of 20 to 40 milligrams; 20 milligrams daily is the recommended dose for most older patients. New studies suggest Celexa also helps prevent recurrence of depression in the elderly.

Celexa and Younger Patients

There have been no studies with Celexa and patients under age 18.

Cost

Celexa costs about 25 percent less than other SSRIs, which according to its manufacturer was a deliberate attempt to make the drug available to as many people as possible.

Who Should Take Celexa Cautiously

People with mania, seizures, liver disease, or severe kidney problems should discuss their condition with their doctor before taking Celexa. Patients with mild kidney problems can take Celexa at a normal dose. Celexa stays in the body twice as long in patients with liver problems, so doses of no more than 20 milligrams are recommended.

Zoloft

This drug has been approved for the treatment of major depression, post-traumatic stress disorder, obsessive-compulsive disorder (OCD), and panic disorder.

No generic version of this drug is available, although its patent expires in 2005, thus paving the way for less expensive alternatives. Zoloft is currently unavailable in liquid form. Most people with depression or OCD begin with a daily dose of 50 milligrams. If there is no improvement after several weeks, your doctor may increase the dosage and reassess your condition after another week or two. Severely depressed individuals may need up to 200 milligrams a day to ease symptoms—but no one should take more than the daily dose. The usual beginning dose for the treatment of panic disorder is 25 milligrams daily, increased to 50 milligrams after the first week if needed; but no more than 200 milligrams daily should be taken.

After the first dose, the drug remains in the body for about 24 hours, but after several days, the drug takes at least 48 hours to leave the body.

The risk of death from overdose is extremely low, as with most SSRIs, but overdoses combined with other drugs or alcohol can sometimes be fatal.

Side Effects

Like most of the SSRIs, Zoloft can cause problems in sexual functioning. While studies put this risk at anywhere between 2 and 17 percent, doctors have in fact found that many patients simply don't report sexual problems in connection with antidepressants. Problems linked to Zoloft include impotence, difficulty reaching orgasm, and lessened sexual desire in general. In some studies, men reported that problems with ejaculation were so troublesome that they stopped taking the drug.

Often, one of the first side effects people notice is tiredness, but this varies from one person to the next. Other medications that cause drowsiness (such as painkillers or antihistamines) may boost the drowsiness you experience with Zoloft.

Other common side effects with Zoloft are insomnia, diarrhea, tremor, and dizziness or lightheadedness. Dry mouth may also appear; if it lasts for more than two weeks, discuss it with your doctor. Nausea or stomach upset may occur but should ease if you take the drug with food or beverages. If it is severe or continues for more than a few days, discuss the problem with your doctor.

Zoloft, like other SSRIs, may also trigger mild mania in some people who already have that tendency. Studies suggest that 4 out of every 1,000 patients experience manic episodes.

Some patients notice a very small weight loss—and appetite loss—with Zoloft. Some studies of patients taking Zoloft for OCD found that 4 out of 1,800 experienced seizures (although clinical trials for depression involving 3,000 patients found no link to seizures with Zoloft). Because higher doses of Zoloft were used to treat OCD, scientists suspect that Zoloft in higher doses may carry a slightly higher risk of seizures.

There have also been rare reports of altered platelet function in patients taking Zoloft, causing abnormal bleeding and purple skin spots. Also, there have been a few very rare cases of low sodium levels, a condition known as "hyponatremia," especially among older people taking Zoloft. Like other problems of the electrolytes, this can be serious when it occurs in the elderly.

Drug Interactions

Research suggests that Zoloft, unlike MAOIs or tricyclics, doesn't necessarily appear to cause problems when mixed with alcohol (but Zoloft's manufacturers don't recommend the combination). There are no known dangerous reactions between nonprescription drugs and Zoloft, but be sure to talk to your doctor about any other drugs you take.

Combining Zoloft with either digitoxin or warfarin (Coumadin) may cause unwanted side effects. And, of course, you should never combine Zoloft or any other SSRI with any MAOI (such as Eldepryl, Furoxone, Matulane, Nardil, and Parnate), because serious (and fatal) reactions have been reported as long as two weeks between the use of Zoloft and one of these drugs. People who have been using Zoloft for more than three months should not take an MAOI (and vice versa) until at least three weeks have passed.

Food Interactions

Unlike most other SSRIs, food affects the blood levels of Zoloft by increasing them approximately 25 percent, although this increase isn't a problem. You can take Zoloft with either food or beverages (and if the drug makes you feel nauseated, taking it with food or milk may help ease the discomfort).

Pregnancy and Breast-feeding

Animal studies suggest that Zoloft may cause developmental problems or decrease survival of offspring. Zoloft was reclassified as pregnancy category C by the FDA when studies showed abnormal effects on the fetus, including stillbirth, decreased birth weight, and perinatal death. However, there have been no human studies with the drug, but based on the animal studies, it's important to weigh the benefits of the drug against the risk to the fetus.

It isn't known if Zoloft is excreted in breast milk.

Zoloft and Older Patients

Studies show that Zoloft is effective among those over age 60, and there are no recommendations for a lower dose in senior citizens. However, older patients with any other medical condition, or those taking many different drugs, may need smaller or less frequent doses of Zoloft upon recommendation of a doctor.

Zoloft and Children

Zoloft is not approved for use in children, but that doesn't mean that doctors don't prescribe it for off label use (a common practice for a wide range of drugs). Not many studies have been done with Zoloft and children.

Cost

The price for Zoloft (whether 25, 50, or 100 milligrams) is about the same, although price will vary from one part of the country to another. In general, expect to pay between $50 and $100 for 30 tablets.

Who Should Take Zoloft Cautiously

Because Zoloft is broken down by the liver, people with even mild cirrhosis or hepatitis should take lower amounts of the drug. Those with severe liver disease should take a drug that is metabolized by the kidneys and not the liver. Patients with liver disease who took Zoloft had much higher blood concentrations of the drug and needed twice as long to rid their bodies of the medication.

Because higher doses of Zoloft have been associated with a slightly higher risk of seizures, patients with a history of seizures or convulsions should be careful taking Zoloft.

People with kidney disease may need smaller doses of Zoloft, but the effects in those with kidney problems hasn't been studied.

Luvox

Luvox (fluvoxamine) was approved by the FDA for the treatment of OCD in adults in December 1994, and for the treatment of OCD in children and adolescents in 1997. First approved for use in Switzerland in 1983, it has already been used to treat thousands of depressed patients in the United States and throughout the world. While not specifically approved as an antidepressant, it is widely prescribed for depression. The patent on the drug expired in 1999.

Most patients are started with a dose between 50 and 100 milligrams taken at bedtime for the first week, and gradually raised to 100 to 200 milligrams. Some people, however, need doses as high as 300 milligrams a day to control their symptoms. A daily dose of more than 100 milligrams should be divided, one in the morning and one at bedtime. Food and milk don't affect the action of the drug, so you may take it with food to ease any nausea or upset stomach.

After the first dose, the drug remains in the body for about 16 hours; after several days it remains for at least 32 hours. Patients should expect to wait between two to four weeks before relief is noticed, although it may take as long as one to two months for symptoms to ease.

The risk of death from overdose of Luvox is considered extremely low when taken alone; there have been only 2 recorded deaths of Luvox overdose, but 17 when Luvox was combined with other drugs.

Side Effects

Luvox, like other SSRIs, can also trigger mild mania in some people with such a tendency. Studies suggest that about 1 percent of those taking the drug experienced mild mania. Other common symptoms include nausea and upset stomach, drowsiness, headache, insomnia, dry mouth, weakness, nervousness, dizziness, diarrhea, constipation, weight loss, or appetite loss.

Luvox also has an effect on some sexual function, including problems reaching orgasm, ejaculation, maintaining erections, impotence, and lack of libido.

In very rare cases (2 out of 1,000), people with a history of seizures taking Luvox for OCD experienced some type of seizure.

Drug Interactions

Never combine Luvox with any MAOI (such as Eldepryl, Nardil, and Parnate), because serious (and fatal) reactions have been reported as long as two weeks between the use of Luvox and an MAOI. You should not start Luvox until at least two weeks have passed after stopping MAOI treatment; if you've used Luvox for more than three months, don't start treatment with the other drug until three weeks have passed.

> ➤ *Warfarin (Coumadin):* increases warfarin blood levels by 98 percent

➤ *Tryptophan:* may produce excessive levels of
   serotonin, causing agitation, restlessness,
   insomnia, anxiety, and stomach problems

➤ *Theophylline:* may increase blood levels of
   drugs containing theophylline

In addition, Luvox may boost the blood levels of a
variety of drugs, including Tegretol, lithium, tricyclic antidepressants, Inderal, Lopressor, methadone, and caffeine.
Luvox and Clozaril may lead to seizures and low blood
pressure. In rare cases, Luvox may cause muscular or
coordination problems when taken with Imitrex.

Pregnancy and Breast-feeding

Animal studies indicate that Luvox may cause developmental problems or decrease survival of offspring. Luvox was
classified as pregnancy category C by the FDA because
studies showed abnormal effects on the fetus, including
stillbirth, decreased birth weight, and perinatal death.
Based on the animal studies, it's important to weigh the
benefits of the drug against the risk to the fetus.

Luvox is excreted in breast milk at about the same
concentrations as the drug found in the mother's blood.
Studies have not been done on the effect of Luvox on
infants; for this reason, mothers should never breast-feed
when taking Luvox.

Luvox and Older Patients

Studies suggest that Luvox is effective in treating depression in people over age 60, but these individuals showed a

40 percent increase in drug concentrations in their blood compared to younger patients.

Luvox and Children

Luvox is the only SSRI formally approved for the treatment of OCD in children. The recommended dose for children ages 8 to 17 is 25 milligrams at bedtime to begin, gradually increased by 25 milligrams per day every four to seven days. A typical dose is between 50 and 200 milligrams daily, and daily doses above 50 milligrams should be divided. The drug is not approved for children under age 8.

Cost

Luvox is slightly less expensive than other SSRIs, although exact prices will differ from one part of the country to another and from pharmacy to pharmacy. On average, 30 tablets of Luvox cost around $65 to $88.

Who Should Take Luvox Cautiously

Anyone with severe liver or kidney disease needs to be careful of the Luvox dosage, since these conditions can keep the drug in the body for as much as 30 percent longer.

Paxil

Paxil (paroxetine) has been approved by the FDA for the treatment of depression, OCD, panic disorder, social anxiety disorder, and generalized anxiety disorder (GAD)—a condition characterized by excessive anxiety and worry about a number of events or activities. The FDA is considering approval of Paxil to treat post-traumatic stress disorder (PTSD).

Results from a multicenter study show that people with GAD experienced nearly a 60 percent reduction in anxiety symptoms when taking Paxil, which also helped reduce tension and disability.

While there is no generic version of this drug, its patent expired in 2000. Paxil is currently not available in liquid form. Most people with depression or OCD start with a dose of 20 milligrams a day. If no improvement occurs over several weeks, the dosage may be increased to 50 milligrams. For panic disorder, patients are usually started at 10 milligrams and gradually raised to no more than 60 milligrams daily.

After the first dose, the drug remains in the body for about 21 hours; after several days, it remains for at least 42 hours. It may take between several weeks to a few months to notice an improvement in symptoms, although patients are often sleeping better within one to two weeks. The risk of overdose is extremely low, like most SSRIs, but overdoses of Paxil combined with other drugs may sometimes be fatal.

Side Effects

Like most of the SSRIs, Paxil can cause problems in sexual functioning, including difficulty reaching orgasm, impotence, and lack of sexual desire. In some studies, men reported that problems with ejaculation were so troublesome that they stopped taking the drug.

While there's no direct evidence that Paxil might cause infertility, a decrease in fertility among male and female rats was observed.

Most other side effects are fairly mild and include tiredness, insomnia, nausea, headache, constipation, weakness, sweating, diarrhea, tremor, and dizziness or lightheadedness. Dry mouth may also appear; discuss this with your doctor if it lasts more than two weeks.

Paxil can also trigger mild mania in some people who already have that tendency. Studies suggest that 4 out of every 1,000 patients experience manic episodes.

Some patients notice a very slight weight loss (and appetite loss) with Paxil, while some notice increased appetite and weight gain. And, in very rare cases, 1 out of 1,800 people on Paxil experienced seizures, according to some studies.

There have also been rare reports of altered platelet function in patients taking Paxil, causing abnormal bleeding and purple skin spots. Also, hyponatremia (low sodium levels—which can be serious when occurring among the elderly) have occurred in rare instances among older people taking Paxil.

In general, most people aren't bothered by side effects enough to stop taking the drug.

Drug Interactions

There are no known dangerous reactions between non-prescription drugs and Paxil, but be sure to talk to your doctor about any other drugs you are taking.

Combining Paxil with warfarin (Coumadin) may cause unwanted side effects. Never combine

Luvox with any MAOI (such as Eldepryl, Nardil, and Parnate), because serious (and fatal) reactions have been reported as long as two weeks between the use of Paxil and an MAOI. People who have been taking Paxil for more than three months should not take an MAOI (and vice versa) until at least three weeks have passed.

> ➤ *Warfarin (Coumadin):* increases warfarin blood levels

> ➤ *Tryptophan:* may produce excessive levels of serotonin, causing agitation, restlessness, insomnia, anxiety, and stomach problems

> ➤ *Dilantin and phenobarbitol:* may decrease blood levels of Paxil

> ➤ *Tagamet:* may increase blood levels of Paxil

In addition, Paxil may boost the blood levels of a variety of drugs, including lithium, theophylline-containing drugs, and Kemadrin. Rarely, Paxil may cause muscular or coordination problems when taken with Imitrex.

Food Interactions

Food doesn't affect the blood levels of Paxil, and you can take it with either food or beverages. If the drug makes you nauseated, taking it with food or milk may help ease the discomfort.

Pregnancy and Breast-feeding

Paxil was classified as pregnancy category C by the FDA indicating a potential problem during pregnancy, but animal studies using doses up to 50 times the maximum dose of Paxil did not appear to harm the fetus. However, when Paxil was given to rats during the third trimester, more of the young rats died within a few days of birth.

Paxil is excreted in breast milk, but levels are considered too small to harm the baby, according to new research. Moreover, the infants had no detectable levels of Paxil in their blood.

Paxil and Older Patients

Studies among people over age 60 indicate that Paxil is effective among this age group. But studies show that concentrations of Paxil among the elderly were 70 to 80 percent higher than in younger patients. For this reason, older patients should start with lower doses.

Paxil and Children

Paxil is not approved for use in children, but that doesn't mean that doctors don't prescribe it for off label use (a common practice for a wide range of drugs).

Cost

Paxil (whether 25, 50, or 100 milligrams) costs between $48 and $90 for 30 tablets, although prices will differ from one part of the country to another.

Who Should Take Paxil Cautiously

Because Paxil is broken down by the liver, people with liver disease (even mild cirrhosis or hepatitis) should take lower amounts of the drug. Those with severe liver disease should take a drug that is metabolized by the kidneys and not the liver. Patients with liver disease who took Paxil had much higher blood concentrations of the drug and needed twice as long to rid their bodies of the medication. People with kidney disease may need smaller doses of Paxil, but the effects in those with kidney problems hasn't been studied.

Conclusion

We've seen how the SSRIs have transformed the treatment of depression by offering a choice of several drugs with low toxicity and few side effects. Unfortunately, not everyone responds to these new drugs; for some people, older antidepressants are far more effective. In chapter 4, we'll explore the structurally unrelated drugs—newer antidepressants that include Wellbutrin, Serzone, Desyrel, Remeron, Effexor, and Vestra.

4 Structurally Unrelated Drugs

"When I was depressed, it was like having a tight metal band around my head all the time. I felt like my cognitive processes couldn't run with the energy they should have. When I took Wellbutrin and my depression lifted, the band loosened and the relief was incredible."

—Jim, 42

Jim was the son of two alcoholics, a brilliant but erratic man who blazed through his adolescence and early adulthood and crashed into a fog of depression in medical school. For the next 10 years, he was haunted by intermittent episodes of depression. But it was his inability to function at work that Jim, a drug company executive, found most troubling.

"The problems my depression was causing me at work were particularly devastating," he recalls today. "I was trying to build my ego late in life, which is fairly common among the children of alcoholics. And my depression was getting in the way of my healthy functioning."

In a vain attempt at self-medication, Jim began using cocaine regularly. When he was finally given a prescription for Wellbutrin, he had given up hope that he would ever regain his ability to think clearly.

Within a week, he began to notice an effect. Within five or six weeks, his depression was gone. "Being able to focus again on work, instead of on myself and my problems, was initially the most uplifting effect," he recalls. Wellbutrin also helped him overcome his cocaine addiction.

Effexor (venlafaxine), Serzone (nefazodone), Remeron (mirtazapine), Desyrel (trazodone), Wellbutrin (bupropion), and Vestra (reboxetine) are a group of structurally unrelated antidepressants that don't fit into any of the established antidepressant drug classes of SSRIs, tricyclics, or MAOIs.

These six are among a group of drugs that scientists have discovered as a result of fiddling with the biochemistry of antidepressants, looking for the perfect medication that's safe, nontoxic, and effective. Only five of the six so far have been approved and are very effective antidepressants, each one affecting a different neurotransmitter system: Effexor affects norepinephrine, serotonin, and dopamine; Serzone boosts serotonin while blocking serotonin receptors; Remeron stimulates norepinephrine and serotonin release as it blocks certain receptors; Desyrel affects serotonin; and Wellbutrin affects norepinephrine and dopamine.

Pros and Cons

Effexor, Serzone, Remeron, Desyrel, and Wellbutrin appear to cause fewer side effects than MAO inhibitors or tricyclics. But because these drugs can cause a few unusual problems in some people, chances are your psychiatrist will be more likely to choose an SSRI like Prozac or Zoloft first.

The most common side effects of the structurally unrelated drugs include agitation, dry mouth, insomnia, sedation, headache, nausea and vomiting, constipation, and tremors.

Effexor (Venlafaxine)

This drug is the first of a new class of structurally novel antidepressants known as "serotonin norepinephrine reuptake inhibitors" (SNRIs). Approved by the FDA in 1994 (with a single-dose version in 1997), Effexor is structurally unlike any other antidepressant; people who don't respond to the SSRIs or one of the tricyclics often do respond to this medication.

Tricia, 39, is a Boston nurse who ended up taking Effexor for lifelong depression after trying every known tricyclic. "The first effects of Effexor were visual," she recalls. "I felt as if there was a cool breeze blowing behind my eyes. Colors were sharper, and all my senses perked up. I feel the way I imagine normal people feel, without struggling through the haze of depression. It clarified things. Before Effexor, every morning I would usually have a few suicidal thoughts before I left for work. Now I'm afraid that this normal feeling will be taken away."

At least one study suggests that Effexor may be more effective than Prozac in treating depression and achieving remission. Published in a February 2000 issue of the *Journal of Affective Disorders,* the study showed that twice as many people treated with Effexor had a full remission when compared to Prozac.

The FDA originally approved Effexor for the treatment of depression, adding a new label change in July 2000 for use as a long-term treatment for generalized anxiety disorder (GAD). Effexor is the first and only antidepressant indicated for both short- and long-term GAD treatment. Because symptoms of GAD persist for many years, Effexor can provide long-term symptom relief from uncontrollable, exaggerated, and persistent worries and anxiety. Nearly 5 percent of Americans have GAD, one of the most common anxiety disorders; nearly two-thirds of patients are women.

New research also suggests that Effexor may be effective in treating symptoms of premenstrual dysphoric disorder (PMDD), a more severe form of premenstrual syndrome (PMS). PMDD affects between 3 to 5 percent of women worldwide and causes severe depression, anxiety, and sudden mood shifts. Although doctors aren't sure what causes PMDD, some believe it may be a complex interaction between ovarian steroids and transmitters in the brain.

Unlike the SSRIs, Prozac, Paxil, Zoloft, Luvox, and Celexa, which only affect serotonin, Effexor interferes with the reuptake of norepinephrine and serotonin and, to a lesser extent, dopamine.

Effexor is excreted by the body in at least 20 hours. Once available only in multiple-dosing regimens, Effexor

XR provides the convenience of once-a-day doses. Most patients begin with 75 milligrams in one daily dose, although some doctors may begin their patients on 37.5 milligrams for four to seven days before increasing the dosage to 75 milligrams. Some patients who don't respond to 75 milligrams per day may respond to a 150-milligram capsule (up to a maximum of 225 milligrams per day). Dose increases are usually taken in increments of 37.5 milligrams a day at intervals not less than every four days. Patients with mild kidney or liver disease may do better on the lower dosage.

You should take Effexor with food or milk to prevent nausea, and since individual doses vary a great deal from one person to the next, pay attention to the directions from your doctor. If you and your doctor decide to discontinue Effexor, you should gradually withdraw as directed.

Side Effects

As with most antidepressants, Effexor can cause dose-related side effects such as nausea; drug-related drowsiness may contribute to impaired thinking, judgment, and motor skills. For this reason, be extra cautious about driving, using machinery, or doing anything that requires alertness, judgment, or physical coordination until you and your doctor feel reasonably confident that the drug won't impair your abilities. Other common symptoms include dry mouth, dizziness, headaches, abnormal ejaculation, loss of appetite, and impotence. Dizziness and nausea usually subside within the first two weeks.

Less frequent side effects include nervousness, insomnia, sweating, and dose-related increases in heart rate (8 beats per minute faster). In general, however, Effexor is well-tolerated and causes fewer side effects than traditional antidepressants. Because Effexor can sometimes cause a spike in blood pressure, your blood pressure should be monitored. Seizures have occasionally been reported.

Withdrawal

Effexor, like SSRIs and tricyclics, can lead to a "discontinuation syndrome" after abruptly stopping the medication. Symptoms include dizziness, dry mouth, insomnia, nausea, nervousness, and sweating. For this reason, if you have taken Effexor for more than one week, you should taper off the dose to minimize the risk of these symptoms. If you've taken the drug for more than six weeks, you should taper off the dose gradually over a two-week period.

Drug Interactions

Never combine Effexor with any monoamine oxidase inhibitor (such as Eldepryl, Nardil, and Parnate) because serious and fatal reactions could occur. Allow at least two weeks between stopping one of these drugs and beginning Effexor. Effexor hasn't been shown to boost the negative effects of alcohol, but patients nevertheless should avoid alcohol when taking this drug.

Ask your pharmacist or doctor about whether Effexor is safe while taking other over-the-counter and/or prescription medication. Unpleasant or hazardous drug interactions are possible. There is a slight chance for an interaction between Effexor and certain drugs, including:

➤ Lithium

➤ Diazepam

➤ Cimetidine (use Effexor and cimetidine with caution if you are elderly or have high blood pressure or liver problems)

➤ Haloperidol (blood levels increase with Effexor by 70 percent)

Pregnancy and Breast-feeding

Effexor is listed as pregnancy category C by the FDA. Animal studies resulted in rat stillbirths, lower rat pup weight, and an increase in pup deaths during the first five days of nursing at two-and-a-half times the maximum human daily dose. The effect of Effexor on labor and delivery is unknown. While there have been no human studies with the drug, it's important to weigh the risk of damage to the fetus against the risk of going without the antidepressant during pregnancy.

Experts don't know if Effexor is found in breast milk; but because many drugs are excreted during breast-feeding, ask your doctor if it's okay to nurse while taking this drug.

Effexor and Older Patients

No change in dosage is necessary in the elderly, although these patients should be treated with caution, since some people may be more sensitive than others.

Effexor and Younger Patients

The safety and effectiveness of Effexor in children under age 18 has not been established.

Who Should Use Effexor Cautiously

Patients with severe kidney or liver disease need lower doses of this medication. Those with moderate kidney problems should reduce the daily dose by 25 percent; but those on kidney dialysis should cut dosage by 50 percent at least four hours after completing dialysis. Patients with moderate liver disease should cut dosage by 50 percent; those with cirrhosis may need even smaller doses.

Serzone (Nefazodone)

When taking Serzone, many people first notice that they start feeling less anxious and can finally get a good night's sleep. As they continue taking Serzone over the next several weeks, the drug steadily relieves the underlying depression while restoring the ability to concentrate. It may take from four to six weeks to really respond to the drug.

Approved in 1994, Serzone was the first of a new type of antidepressant with a chemical structure unrelated to SSRIs, tricyclics, tetracyclics, or MAOIs. Combining the primary mechanisms of the SSRIs and the tricyclics, it's actually more similar to the tricyclics in action. Its ability to help people sleep may make it helpful for depressed people who are also anxious or agitated or who struggle with insomnia. In addition, Serzone causes fewer cases of sexual dysfunction—a problem that occurs in as many as

40 to 70 percent of patients on antidepressants. Serzone has an incidence of sexual problems at just 1.5 percent, according to its manufacturer Bristol-Myers.

How it works exactly is unknown, but studies suggest that Serzone interferes with the uptake of both serotonin and norepinephrine and can produce some dramatic improvements in depression. It's the first drug to boost the brain's level of serotonin while blocking serotonin receptors. While clinical trials found Serzone to be as effective at easing depression as other drugs, when taken twice daily it shows little tendency to disturb sleep. (This is important since as many as one in five people taking an SSRI must also take some type of prescription sleep aid.)

The recommended initial dose ranges between 150 and 300 milligrams per day in divided doses. An effective dose is usually between 300 and 600 milligrams daily; but don't take more than 600 milligrams a day. Seniors and people with kidney or liver problems may require lower doses.

Serzone reaches optimum blood levels in four to five days with twice daily dosing. After stopping the drug, it is almost completely eliminated from the body within five days.

Side Effects

Possible Serzone side effects include dry mouth (25 percent), drowsiness (25 percent), nausea (22 percent), dizziness (17 percent), constipation (14 percent), weakness (11 percent), lightheadedness (10 percent), blurred vision (9 percent), and confusion (7 percent).

If you are male and experience a prolonged or inappropriate erection while taking Serzone, discontinue this drug and call your doctor.

Drug Interactions

If Serzone is taken with certain drugs, the effects of either may be increased, decreased, or altered. Serzone cannot be taken with MAOIs. It should not be given at the same time as triazolam (Halcion) or aprazolam (Xanax) because it significantly increases the blood concentrations of these medications. It can also cause more drowsiness than an SSRI would, although the effect decreases with continued use. It is especially important to check with your doctor before combining Serzone with the following:

➤ Alcohol

➤ Digoxin (Lanoxin)

Pregnancy and Breast-feeding

The effects of Serzone during pregnancy have not been adequately studied. If you are pregnant or are planning to become pregnant, tell your doctor immediately. Serzone should only be used during pregnancy if clearly needed.

Because Serzone may appear in breast milk, your doctor may tell you to discontinue breast-feeding if this medication is essential to your health.

Serzone and Older Patients

Older people (especially women) should start with half the usual dose of Serzone because they may have more trouble breaking down this drug in their bodies. The usual starting dose for older or sick patients is 100 milligrams a day taken in two doses.

Serzone and Younger Patients

Serzone has not been studied in patients under the age of 18.

Who Should Use Serzone Cautiously

Serzone should be used cautiously in patients with a history of mania or heart or liver disease. Because it may lower the seizure threshold, it should never be used in patients with a known seizure disorder. It should also be used with caution by those who have had a heart attack or stroke or who suffer from dehydration.

Remeron (Mirtazapine)

Approved by the FDA in 1996, Remeron offers another approach to the treatment of depression and is often helpful in treating insomnia or anxiety. Remeron does not broadly block the reuptake of norepinephrine or serotonin like the SSRIs do. Instead, Remeron stimulates the release of norepinephrine and serotonin, while blocking two specific serotonin receptors that have been linked with lowered sex drive, nausea, nervousness, headache, insomnia, and diarrhea. As a result, Remeron typically does not cause any of these side effects, nor does it appear to have a harmful effect on the heart—even at 22 times the maximum recommended dose. Loss of sexual interest or ability—a typical side effect of SSRIs—was a problem for only 1 percent of depressed patients on Remeron. This ability to target specific serotonin receptors marks the next significant advance in the evolution of biochemical selectivity of antidepressants.

"I didn't think I'd ever feel this good again," said Joe, a 43-year-old severely depressed teacher who had tried several other antidepressants without success. "I even got my sex life back!"

Your doctor will probably start you off with 15 milligrams a day. If this isn't effective, the dose may be increased every one to two weeks to allow sufficient time for the effectiveness of the dose to be evaluated. The maximum recommended dose is 45 milligrams a day.

You can take Remeron with or without food, preferably in the evening before going to sleep. Even though you may begin to feel better in one to four weeks, continue taking the drug exactly as prescribed. Regular daily doses are needed for the drug to work properly.

Side Effects

While Remeron avoids many of the common side effects of other antidepressants, it is still not free of all side effects. The most common complaints are weight gain (12 percent) and temporary sleepiness (54 percent), which is less frequent at higher doses. Other side effects are increased appetite (17 percent) and dizziness (7 percent). About 15 percent reported higher cholesterol readings with this drug. (If you have a cholesterol problem, be sure to mention this to your doctor before starting Remeron.) Other problems may include abnormal dreams and thinking, constipation, dry mouth, flulike symptoms, and weakness.

Less common side effects may include back pain, confusion, difficult or labored breathing, fluid retention, frequent urination, muscle pain, nausea, swelling of the ankles or hands, or tremors. When first taking this medication, you may feel dizzy or lightheaded, especially when getting up from a lying or sitting position. If standing up slowly doesn't help, or if this problem continues, inform your doctor.

One rare but unpleasant side effect is agranulocytosis, a condition in which the blood marrow becomes damaged so that white blood cells can't be produced. Since white blood cells are crucial to the body's immune system, this can be fatal if untreated. However, once the patient stops taking the drug, the condition reverses itself. Although rare, the risk of this condition may make some doctors reluctant to prescribe Remeron. *Warning: Consult your doctor immediately if you develop a sore throat, fever, inflamed mucous membranes of the mouth, or other signs of infection when taking Remeron.*

Withdrawal

You shouldn't abruptly stop taking antidepressants as withdrawal effects may occur. Suddenly going off the drug may also cause the recurrence of depressive symptoms. Speak to your doctor about slowly tapering off the drug.

Drug Interactions

As with SSRIs, you should not take Remeron with any monoamine oxidase inhibitor (MAOI) or use it within two weeks of stopping or starting MAOI treatment. Remeron is metabolized by the liver and its effect on the metabolism of other drugs is not yet clearly known. If Remeron is taken with certain drugs, the effects of either may be increased, decreased, or altered. It is especially important to check with your doctor before combining Remeron with tranquilizers such as Valium, Xanax, and Ativan.

Pregnancy and Breast-feeding

The effects of Remeron during pregnancy have not been adequately studied. If you are pregnant or planning to become pregnant, tell your doctor immediately. Because Remeron may appear in breast milk, also tell your doctor if you plan to breast-feed.

Remeron and Older Patients

Older people (especially men) may find that it takes longer for the drug to clear the body. Because they are more sensitive to antidepressant drugs, older patients may find smaller doses satisfactory.

Remeron and Younger Patients

The safety and effectiveness of Remeron has not been established in children.

Who Should Use Remeron Cautiously

Remeron should be used with caution by anyone with heart, blood pressure, liver, or kidney problems. Seniors and people with kidney and liver problems may require lower doses. Be sure to tell your doctor if you have a

history of seizures, mania (extremely high spirits), hypomania (mild excitability), drug use, or any other physical
or emotional problems.

Desyrel (Trazodone)

This novel antidepressant is chemically unrelated to tricyclic, tetracyclic, or other antidepressants. How Desyrel
works is not fully understood, but it is believed to inhibit
serotonin uptake.

Desyrel should be taken with food or shortly after
a meal or light snack to lower the risk of dizziness or
lightheadedness. You may be more apt to feel dizzy or
lightheaded if you take the drug before you have eaten.
The recommended initial dose is 150 milligrams daily.
This may be increased every few days by 50 milligrams a
day to a maximum daily dose of 600 milligrams. Once
you have responded well to Desyrel, your doctor may
gradually reduce your dose.

Side Effects

Unlike antidepressants such as Prozac that may leave you
pacing the floor at night, Desyrel can have you sleeping
like a baby. Because of Desyrel's sedative qualities, it's
often added to other drugs such as Prozac if insomnia
becomes problematic.

On the downside, Desyrel may cause a rare but nasty
side effect called priapism, a painful erection without sexual arousal. Priapism occurs when blood doesn't drain
from the penis's spongy tissue, keeping it erect. Urgent
treatment is needed in this case because of the risk of

permanent damage to the penis. (Some patients have experienced permanent impairment of erection or impotence.) Desyrel has also been linked to some heart problems.

Other side effects include dry mouth (34 percent), dizziness (28 percent), blurred vision (15 percent), and nausea (13 percent).

You may need to undergo blood tests since this drug can reduce your white blood cell count. (White blood cells are an important part of the body's immune system; low levels could be a problem if you develop an infection, sore throat, or fever.) Because of the link between Desyrel and some heart problems, your doctor may ask you to have blood pressure readings and electrocardiograms.

If you get too sleepy or dizzy, ask your doctor if you can take a larger portion of your total dose at bedtime, dividing the rest into two or three smaller doses during the day. Be extra cautious about driving, using machinery, or engaging in any activities that require alertness, judgment, or physical coordination until you and your doctor feel reasonably confident that the drug does not impair your abilities.

Drug Interactions

If Desyrel is taken with certain drugs, the effects of either may be increased, decreased, or altered. Desyrel may intensify the effects of alcohol, so you should not combine it with alcoholic beverages. It is especially important to check with your doctor before combining Desyrel with any of the following:

➤ Barbiturates such as Seconal

➤ Central nervous system depressants such as Demerol or Halcion

➤ Chlorpromazine (Thorazine)

➤ Digoxin (Lanoxin)

➤ Drugs for high blood pressure such as Catapres and Wytensin

➤ Other antidepressants such as Prozac and Norpramin

➤ Phenytoin (Dilantin)

➤ Warfarin (Coumadin)

Little is known about the interaction between Desyrel and general anesthetics; therefore, this drug should be discontinued prior to elective surgery.

Pregnancy and Breast-feeding

Because some animal studies have revealed fetal deaths and birth defects, Desyrel is not recommended during the first three months of pregnancy. The effects of Desyrel during human pregnancy have not been adequately studied. You and your doctor should weigh the potential risks to the fetus and to you before deciding whether or not to take antidepressants during pregnancy.

Desyrel may appear in breast milk (it has been found in lactating rats). If this drug is essential to your health, your doctor may advise you to discontinue breast-feeding until your treatment is finished.

Desyrel and Older Patients

Because they are more sensitive to antidepressant drugs, older patients may find smaller doses satisfactory.

Desyrel and Younger Patients

The safety and effectiveness of Desyrel has not been established in children under age 18.

Who Should Use Desyrel Cautiously

Desyrel should be used with caution in people with heart disease because it can cause irregular heart beats.

Wellbutrin (Bupropion)

Wellbutrin (bupropion hydrochloride) is an antidepressant that is chemically unrelated to tricyclic, tetracyclic, or other antidepressants. Instead, it is a weak serotonin and norepinephrine reuptake inhibitor that also affects the neurotransmitter dopamine. The actual mechanism is not known.

One of the most demoralizing problems with almost all antidepressants is their negative effect on sexual function, including decreased libido, erection problems, and impotence; and it is often one of the main reasons why people stop taking their antidepressants. Wellbutrin is the drug of choice if other antidepressants cause sexual problems. (It also doesn't cause weight gain or sedation.)

Wellbutrin's boost to the libido can be a welcome relief to many people; indeed, a few find Wellbutrin too sexually stimulating. "I was thinking about sex all the time," complains Hillary, 39, who was given Wellbutrin when Zoloft did not relieve her depression. "I spent all my time in bed."

Typical first dose is 150 milligrams once a day. After about four days, the dosage may be increased to 300 milligrams daily, divided into two or three doses with at least four hours between doses. Wellbutrin is virtually eliminated from the body in about four or five days after the last dose. The maximum allowable dose is 450 milligrams daily in divided doses. To avoid the risk of seizure, no single dose should exceed 200 milligrams.

Dosage should be increased slowly to avoid agitation and insomnia. Timing the last dose after the evening meal rather than at bedtime can minimize insomnia.

Generic versions of bupropion may soon be available.

Other Uses of Wellbutrin

Under the name Zyban, bupropion is FDA-approved to help smokers kick the habit, while limiting the weight gain for those who have stopped smoking. It is unknown how Zyban works to help people stop smoking, but some experts think that since the drugs increase neurotransmitters in the brain, it may somehow interfere with nicotine use at this level.

Recently, Wellbutrin has been used with some success to treat attention deficit/hyperactivity disorder (ADHD), although this use has not been approved by the FDA.

Side Effects

Common side effects at 300 milligrams include dry mouth (17 percent), nausea (13 percent), insomnia (11 percent), dizziness (7 percent), and sore throat (3 percent). At high doses it can cause anxiety, high blood pressure, and seizures—especially among those with eating disorders such as bulimia and anorexia. Other side effects include agitation, headache/migraine, constipation, tremor, or hallucinations.

Some patients find that Wellbutrin's actions on the central nervous system can produce unpleasant hypersensitivity. "When I took Wellbutrin, I spent a lot of time on my sofa with the blankets over my head," comments Eleanor, a 39-year-old stockbroker. "I felt oversensitized all over my body. It just felt weird."

Because Wellbutrin blocks dopamine, this drug may also rarely produce movement disorders and changes in the endocrine system.

"Wellbutrin is usually my second-choice antidepressant," says psychiatrist Andy Myerson. "I've had remarkable success with it, but many people are scared by the potential for seizures. It's tricky."

The biggest problem associated with Wellbutrin is that the risk of seizure is four times higher than with other antidepressants. Overdosing is a particular danger, since the chance of seizure increases almost tenfold at twice the normal daily dose of 300 milligrams. The biggest risk of seizure appears to be in patients who have had a prior serious head injury, prior seizures, brain or spinal cord tumors, those on antiseizure medication, or those whose dosage is suddenly increased. You can lower the risk if you never abruptly increase your dosage, don't take more than 450 milligrams daily, and limit any single dose to no more than 200 milligrams.

A newer formulation of Wellbutrin (Wellbutrin SR) carries a much lower risk of seizure than does the original version.

While there have been no reports that Wellbutrin causes liver damage in humans, animal studies have revealed a variety of liver problems with this drug.

Restlessness is a major problem; anxiety and insomnia (especially at the beginning of treatment) is often a concern with this drug. Some people need to be treated with sedatives or hypnotic drugs to ease their anxiety. (Wellbutrin SR has a more favorable side effect profile than the original version.)

Although Wellbutrin occasionally causes weight gain, a more common effect is weight loss; 28 percent lose 5 pounds or more. If depression has already caused you to lose weight and if further weight loss would be detrimental to your health, this may not be the best antidepressant for you.

Drug Interactions

You should not take Wellbutrin if you are taking an MAOI, or any other drug that contains bupropion (such as Zyban, the smoking cessation product). Do not drink alcohol while taking Wellbutrin; in addition to aggravating drowsiness, alcohol increases the risk of seizures.

If Wellbutrin is taken with certain drugs, the effects of either may be increased, decreased, or altered. It is especially important to check with your doctor before combining Wellbutrin with any of the following:

➤ Tricyclics

➤ Phenytoin (Dilantin)

➤ Levodopa (Larodopa)

➤ Tranquilizers such as Thorazine and Mellaril

➤ Phenobarbital (Luminal)

➤ Tagamet

➤ Tegretol

Pregnancy and Breast-feeding

It's not clear if Wellbutrin is safe during pregnancy, although animal studies did cause birth defects in doses of up to 45 times the human daily dose.

It is not recommended for nursing mothers because Wellbutrin may pass into breast milk and cause serious reactions in a baby. If you are a new mother, you may need to discontinue breast-feeding while taking this medication.

Wellbutrin and Older Patients

Because they are more sensitive to antidepressant drugs, older patients may tolerate smaller doses better.

Wellbutrin and Younger Patients

The safety and effectiveness of Wellbutrin has not been established in children under age 18.

Who Should Use Wellbutrin Cautiously

You should not take Wellbutrin if you currently have any type of seizure disorder, since this drug is associated with a higher risk of seizures, especially at higher doses. At the recommended daily dose of 300 milligrams, the risk of seizures is 0.1 percent (about the same rate as other antidepressants), but at 400 milligrams, the risk rises to 0.4 percent. Avoid this drug if you have bulimia or anorexia (current or prior) since you may have a higher risk of seizures on this drug.

Vestra (Reboxetine)

Vestra (reboxetine), a selective norepinephrine reuptake inhibitor (SNRI) manufactured by Upjohn, received an FDA approval letter in July 1999, but it has not yet received marketing approval. Edronax (another form of reboxetine) is used for the treatment of depression.

SNRIs have been marketed in the United Kingdom since 1997 and in Europe since 1998, where the class is known as NARI (noradrenaline reuptake inhibitor). This class of antidepressants targets noradrenaline. Some depressed people have low levels of this neurochemical, and the SNRIs prevent cells from reabsorbing noradrenaline, boosting its supply in the brain.

While serotonin plays a vital role in mood, noradrenaline is also important in maintaining human drive and the capacity for reward. Drugs that selectively affect noradrenaline appear to help restore a person's energy and motivation.

Side Effects

Reboxetine's side effects include dry mouth, constipation, insomnia, increased sweating, rapid heartbeat, vertigo, urinary hesitance or retention, and impotence (in patients treated with doses above 8 milligrams a day).

Drug Interactions

Avoid using reboxetine with MAOIs. It should also be used cautiously with drugs known to lower blood pressure.

Pregnancy and Breast-feeding

There are no adequate and well-controlled studies in pregnant women, so reboxetine should be used only if the potential benefit to the mother justifies the potential risk to the fetus. Reboxetine is not recommended for women who are breast-feeding.

Who Should Use Vestra Cautiously

Since rare cases of seizures have been reported in clinical studies, patients with a history of convulsive disorders should be closely supervised and should discontinue reboxetine if they develop seizures. Combined usage of MAOIs and reboxetine should be avoided. As with all antidepressants, switches to mania have occurred, and close supervision of bipolar patients is recommended. Patients with urinary retention or glaucoma should also be cautious about taking reboxetine.

Conclusion

In this chapter, we've focused on six new drugs that are unrelated to each other or to any of the earlier classes of antidepressants. In the next chapter, we'll discuss cyclic antidepressants, including the tricyclics and tetracyclics.

5 CYCLIC ANTIDEPRESSANTS

"What I remember most about being depressed was always being exhausted. I could never get to sleep at night, and when I did, I had nightmares. Then I'd wake up in the morning and have to drag myself to work. And in all that time—four or five years, I guess—I never once enjoyed anything. I was actually planning my own suicide when my doctor referred me to a psychiatrist who put me on imipramine. For the first time in years, I finally began to get some pleasure out of life."

—Sam, 43

Before the SSRIs, tricyclics were the first line of defense against encroaching depression, and had been ever since imipramine's release in 1958 under the brand name Tofranil. Today, tricyclics are a less popular choice than the new generation of antidepressants, but they're still an important weapon in the antidepressant arsenal for a subset of people who don't respond to anything else.

Before tricyclics were developed, psychiatrists treating severely depressed clients had only two real choices: amphetamines or electroshock therapy. Imipramine was

COMMON CYCLIC ANTIDEPRESSANTS
(Lower doses are used with elderly patients)

DRUG	USUAL EFFECTIVE DAILY DOSE
Amitriptyline (Elavil, Endep, Emitrip, Enovil)	150–300 mg
Amoxapine (Asendin)	150–400 mg
Clomipramine (Anafranil)	100–150 mg
Desipramine (Norpramin, Pertofrane)	100–300 mg
Doxepin (Adapin, Sinequan)	75–300 mg
Imipramine (Janimine, Tipramine, Tofranil, Tofranil-PM)	150–300 mg
Maprotiline (Ludiomil)	75–150 mg
Nortriptyline (Pamelor, Aventyl)	50–150 mg
Protriptyline (Vivactil)	15–60 mg
Trimipramine (Surmontil)	75–150 mg

discovered by Swiss scientists searching for a successful schizophrenia treatment; it turned out that imipramine didn't do much for schizophrenia at all. What it *did* do very well was perk up depressed patients.

With the discovery of imipramine, doctors finally had a drug that relieved a person's underlying depression. And when scientists realized how effective imipramine was—about 70 percent of depressed patients responded to this drug—they flocked to the laboratories in search of similar drugs based on imipramine's three-ring ("tricyclic") antihistaminic chemical structure. Before long, laboratories all over the country began churning out tricyclic clones, each one a little different from, but none any better than, imipramine itself. A later-developed drug in this class, maprotiline (Ludiomil), had four rings and was therefore called "tetracyclic." Taken together, the tricyclics and tetracyclics are known as "heterocyclics" or "cyclics."

But while all these cyclics were effective, not one provided the perfect solution to depression for which scientists had been searching.

How Cyclic Antidepressants Work

The cyclic antidepressants work by beefing up the brain's supply of norepinephrine and serotonin levels—chemicals that are abnormally low in depressed patients. This allows the flow of nerve impulses to return to normal. The cyclics do *not* act by stimulating the central nervous system or by blocking monoamine oxidase.

The problem with cyclics is that they don't stop there. They go on to interfere with a range of other neurotransmitter systems and a variety of brain cell receptors, affecting nerve cell communication all over the brain in the process. And the more neurotransmitter systems and receptors you affect, the more side effects a patient will have.

Prime Candidates

Side effects notwithstanding, for some people the cyclics work better than any other drug available.

"I've been taking imipramine for the past five years," says Carol, 47, a New Jersey teacher. "It was the first and only antidepressant I've ever taken. When I was depressed, I had a feeling of being lost. I was discontented with myself—I felt 'blah' for a long time. I just don't feel that way anymore."

The challenge, of course, is to figure out *who* will respond best to them. The important thing to understand is that some types of tri- and tetracyclics are riskier than others, and some people tolerate some types better.

Just as scientists aren't sure exactly what causes depression, they're not sure exactly what cures it, either. Often, your doctor will choose an antidepressant drug for you based not on the cause of your depression as much as the symptoms you have, and how well you might be expected to tolerate certain side effects.

Unfortunately, there's no simple test that can reveal which drug might work best for you. How well you react to any particular drug is often as much a surprise to your doctor as it is to you. That's why it may take some time before you and your doctor discover the perfect antidepressant "fit."

The tricyclic nortriptyline (Pamelor), for example, may be useful in treating patients with depression following a stroke.

Both trimipramine and imipramine work equally well at relieving depression in hospitalized patients. Because it has a sedative effect, the tetracyclic Ludiomil is useful in treating depression accompanied by anxiety or sleeping problems. Protriptyline is more likely to aggravate agitation and anxiety, but it's particularly good if you're withdrawn or lethargic and tired. On the other hand, it's likely to cause sleeping problems, especially when taken late in the day. (For this reason, protriptyline is a popular choice in the treatment of narcolepsy.)

In the past, depressed patients were almost always started out on tricyclics. With the growing popularity of SSRIs, however, most patients are now given Prozac or Zoloft, and then moved to a tricyclic or tetracyclic if the depression doesn't respond to the first- or second-choice drugs.

"When I became very depressed after experiencing some family problems, I tried Prozac," reports Gina, 52, a personnel manager in Arizona. "But after six months it hadn't affected my depression at all. So my doctor switched me to imipramine. Within a few weeks, I felt less prone to tears, less hopeless. It's not so much that I was suddenly pro-life. It's just that the negative outlook wasn't so stupefying."

Sometimes, doctors may add Prozac or lithium to small doses of tri- or tetracyclics to boost the antidepressants' effectiveness. However, this can be risky; the combination has sometimes caused an increase in the blood level of the cyclic. Since cyclics already can be dangerous to the heart and can set off seizures, adding Prozac may increase this risk.

Who Shouldn't Take Cyclics

The first job for your doctor is to decide whether you're one of the people who *shouldn't* take cyclic antidepressants (see box, "Complicating Medical Problems"). Obviously, your doctor won't prescribe them if you're allergic to this type of antidepressant. If you've taken an MAOI within the past two weeks, you'll want to wait two weeks before taking cyclics, since the combination of these two can cause serious side effects.

If you have any kind of drinking problem, you should avoid cyclics, since alcohol can be toxic when mixed with these drugs.

Schizophrenics or manic-depressives should only use cyclics with great caution, since these drugs can worsen the symptoms of schizophrenia and may push a depressed manic-depressive into a manic state if the person isn't already taking an anti-manic medication (such as lithium).

There are also some specific health problems that don't mix well with certain antidepressants. If you have a problem with your bone marrow function or any blood cell disorder, or if you have seizures or an adrenalin-producing tumor, you'll want to stay away from clomipramine (Anafranil).

If you have serious heart disease, you should avoid trimipramine (Surmontil). Ludiomil shouldn't be used if you have a seizure disorder, or if you've had a heart attack within the past six weeks.

COMPLICATING MEDICAL PROBLEMS

Before taking cyclic antidepressants, be sure to tell your doctor if you have any of the following medical problems:

➤ Alcohol abuse (cyclics may increase depressant effects of alcohol)
➤ Allergies (to cyclics, to maprotiline or trazodone, foods, preservatives, dyes)
➤ Asthma
➤ Blood disorders
➤ Contact lenses
➤ Convulsions or seizures
➤ Glaucoma or increased eye pressure
➤ Heart disease
➤ High blood pressure
➤ Intestinal problems (cyclics may cause increased risk of serious side effects)
➤ Kidney disease
➤ Liver disease (may raise blood levels of cyclics, causing more side effects)
➤ Manic-depression
➤ Prostate enlargement
➤ Schizophrenia (cyclics may worsen schizophrenia)
➤ Stomach problems (cyclics may cause increased risk of serious side effects)
➤ Thyroid overactivity
➤ Urinary problems

You should also avoid Ludiomil if you have glaucoma or if you're an alcoholic. Also, before giving Ludiomil, your doctor will want to know if you have an enlarged prostate, stomach or intestinal problems, overactive thyroid, asthma, seizure disorders, or liver disease.

How to Use Cyclics

If your doctor is considering one of the cyclics to treat your depression, you may be asked to get a physical examination, an electrocardiogram (EKG), and routine blood tests first. These can help determine which type of drug will be safest for you to use.

No matter which cyclic you take, you'll begin with a small dose, gradually increasing in strength until your depression begins to improve. If you're one of those people who responds well to cyclics, you'll probably notice your sleeping problems improving within the first several days.

Some cyclics may work more quickly than others. A few people find that their depression disappears overnight—they go to sleep feeling depressed and wake up in a completely different mood. Others find their symptoms gradually fade over a period of days.

Don't get discouraged if you're not turning handsprings within moments of starting therapy. Some people find it takes as long as three or four weeks before they see improvement.

Within a month, you'll probably notice that you're starting to be more interested in your surroundings, in other people, and in activities you once enjoyed. As the days pass, you should begin to feel better and better.

"When I began taking imipramine, I thought it would be like taking an aspirin—you pop it in and within an hour you feel different," says Carol. "It didn't happen that way. I began to feel gradual changes by the end of the second week, and by the third week there was quite a difference in my depression."

If you don't respond to a cyclic, it may mean that your dose isn't high enough. Your doctor may order blood tests to find out how much of the drug is actually circulating in your blood, especially if you're taking imipramine, desipramine, nortriptyline, or amitriptyline. If after increasing the dose you still feel depressed after four or five weeks, your doctor will probably switch you to a different drug.

How Cyclics Are Administered

The usual adult dosage of protriptyline is 15 to 40 milligrams daily, divided into three or four doses. If necessary, doses may be increased up to 60 milligrams daily, but doses above this limit are not recommended. Any increases in amount should be given in the morning dose. Lower doses are recommended for adolescents and the elderly.

Your doctor will probably begin with about 75 milligrams of trimipramine daily in divided doses, increasing to 150 milligrams per day. Doses over 200 milligrams daily aren't recommended. Because this drug is so sedating, you can take the entire dose at bedtime.

Ludiomil may be taken in a single daily dose (usually at bedtime) or in divided daily doses. An initial dosage of 75 milligrams daily is usually effective. However, in some patients (such as the elderly, who tend to be oversensitive to antidepressants), an initial dose of 25 milligrams daily is recommended.

Because Ludiomil doesn't break down rapidly in the body, the initial dose should be maintained for at least two weeks. It may then be increased by 25-milligram increments as tolerated. Most people find that a maximum level of 150 milligrams is enough to keep symptoms under control. A maximum of 225 milligrams daily may be needed.

If you're taking Ludiomil for an extended period of time, your doctor may order blood cell counts and liver function studies and may monitor your blood pressure.

An overdose of a cyclic antidepressant may cause hallucinations, drowsiness, enlarged pupils, respiratory failure, fever, irregular heartbeat, severe dizziness, severe muscle stiffness or weakness, restlessness or agitation, breathing problems, vomiting, convulsions, and coma.

IF YOU FORGET A DOSE

One daily dose (bedtime)

➤ *Don't* take a missed bedtime dose in the morning, you may notice uncomfortable side effects during the day.
➤ Check with your doctor about getting back on the correct schedule.

More than one daily dose

➤ If you miss a dose, take the missed dose as soon as possible.
➤ If your missed dose is within an hour of the next one, skip the missed dose and get back on your regular dosage schedule.
➤ *Don't* double doses without your doctor's approval.

These drugs can be dangerous at fairly small amounts (10 to 15 times your normal dose)—and even smaller amounts in children.

Dietary Restrictions

There are some dietary cautions to keep in mind with specific cyclics. If you're taking the liquid version of doxepin (Adapin, Sinequan), don't mix it with grape juice or carbonated beverages, since these may reduce its effectiveness. Mix up this drug just before you take it.

Tolerance

While long-term treatment with antidepressants is controversial, more and more people are taking antidepressants for longer periods. Perhaps as a result, more and more of the antidepressants (even including some of the SSRIs, such as Prozac) are developing a reputation for decreasing effectiveness as treatment progresses.

This is known as tolerance, and among the tricyclics, amoxapine in particular has been associated with this problem. Once you develop tolerance to an antidepressant, you'll need higher doses in order to keep your depression under control.

Side Effects

On the whole, cyclics are pretty safe and effective, falling somewhere between the MAOIs, which have many side effects, and SSRIs, which have very few. Even if you do run into some unpleasant side effects in the beginning, chances are they will become less of a problem as time goes by. If not, you can always switch to a drug with a different side-effect profile.

Side effects with cyclics may include dry mouth, constipation, blurred vision, weight gain, increased heart rate, drowsiness, urinary retention, impotence, decreased blood pressure, and dizziness when standing up. Those with the highest probability for these side effects include amitriptyline, clomipramine, doxepin, imipramine, and trimipramine. Desipramine has the lowest risk for these effects (see box on pages 152 to 153, "Potential Side Effects with Cyclic Antidepressants"). And patients taking high doses of cyclics often complain of memory problems and trouble in finding the right words.

And like every other antidepressant, cyclics can trigger a mild manic high in some people. In a retrospective study published in the *British Medical Journal* of 3,065 patients with major depression, tricyclics worsened suicidal thinking slightly more than Prozac did (16.3 percent compared with 15.3 percent). Suicidal acts were reported as 0.3 percent for Prozac and 0.4 percent for tricyclics.

About 15 percent of people may feel nauseated (compared with about 21 percent of people taking SSRIs); headaches occur in about 20 percent of people taking either SSRIs or tricyclics.

Because some of these drugs are known for sedative effects that cause drowsiness, dizziness, or decreased alertness, don't drive, fly an aircraft, operate dangerous machinery, or do anything requiring alertness until you learn how your medicine affects you.

Dry Mouth, Blurred Vision. As part of their action on many different brain systems, the cyclics act on histamine receptors, flicking on the body's "fight or flight" response, speeding up the heart, and shunting energy away from bodily functions, such as waste removal. The result is dry mouth, blurred vision, constipation, and urinary problems. These side effects may be especially annoying if you're taking amitriptyline, clomipramine, doxepin, imipramine, or protriptyline.

"When I was taking imipramine, I had to chew gum all the time if I wanted to talk," remembers Gail, 52. "And I had to be sure I ate a jar of prunes every day—or else!" She notes that her dry mouth and constipation lasted for the entire two years she took imipramine.

If you're particularly bothered with a dry mouth, you can try sucking on sugarless candy or gum. (A lack of saliva can lead to tooth decay, so try not to aggravate this situation with sugar.) Or ask your physician to prescribe a saliva-promoting drug like pilocarpine.

Blood Sugar Levels. If you're a diabetic, you should be aware that cyclic antidepressants may affect your blood sugar levels. This means that you could notice your blood or urine test results are changing. If you have any questions, check with your doctor.

Constipation. It's important to remember that constipation may be a symptom of your depression and not a side effect of a cyclic antidepressant. If it is a symptom of your depression, the problem should disappear as the cyclic takes effect.

POTENTIAL SIDE EFFECTS WITH
CYCLIC ANTIDEPRESSANTS

COMMON SIDE EFFECTS

- Tremor
- Unpleasant taste
- Dry mouth
- Nausea
- Fatigue
- Weakness
- Anxiety
- Diarrhea
- Headache
- Sensitivity to sunlight
- Constipation
- Indigestion
- Insomnia
- Sedation
- Nervousness
- Excessive sweating

INFREQUENT ADVERSE EFFECTS

- Shakiness
- Vomiting
- Eye pain
- Slow pulse
- Jaundice
- Joint pain
- Fever
- Chills
- Visual changes
- Muscle aches
- Nasal congestion
- Difficult and/or frequent urination
- Dizziness
- Abnormal dreams
- Diminished sex drive
- Inflamed tongue
- Hair loss
- Abdominal pain
- Rash
- Palpitations
- Hiccups
- Back pain
- Irregular heartbeat
- Fainting

RARE ADVERSE EFFECTS

- Itchy skin
- Swollen testicles
- Swollen breasts
- Involuntary movements of jaw, lips, and tongue
- Sore throat
- Nightmares
- Confusion

POTENTIAL SIDE EFFECTS WITH
CYCLIC ANTIDEPRESSANTS *(continued)*

SIDE EFFECTS MORE COMMON
TO PEOPLE OVER AGE 60
- Seizures   ➤ Dizziness
- Headache   ➤ Shaking
- Fainting   ➤ Insomnia
- Urination problems ➤ Hallucinations

If it's clear that you're constipated as a result of the drug, there are some dietary changes you can try. Begin by eating more fruits and vegetables, getting lots of fiber, and drinking plenty of fluids. If all other methods fail, your doctor can prescribe a stool softener or bulk agent. Finally, your doctor can switch you to an antidepressant that carries less of a risk for this type of side effect, such as Prozac or Zoloft or another of the newer antidepressants.

Contact Lenses. You may experience problems with your contact lenses if you take cyclics. Because these drugs can cause dry eyes, your lenses may get gummed up with deposits of thick secretions, making them feel gritty, itchy, or painful. If this happens, your doctor may be able to prescribe a different antidepressant, reduce your dose, or prescribe artificial tears.

Dizziness. Some tricyclics, especially amitriptyline, might make you dizzy when you stand up (this is called "orthostatic hypotension"). If you notice this, try standing up more slowly. In the morning, dangle your feet over the side of the bed for a few minutes before slowly standing up. If you have a serious problem with dizziness, your doctor may be able to adjust your dose or switch you to another cyclic. The tricyclics least likely to cause this problem are amoxapine and nortriptyline (Pamelor).

Drowsiness. Sedation is a common side effect of many tricyclics and tetracyclics; three of the most sedating are doxepin, amitriptyline, and trimipramine.

"I found the sleepiness to be fairly pleasant," Sally, 52, reports. "I was sleepy all the time, but it was a blissful sort of sleepiness. And since I'd been having trouble sleeping before I started taking imipramine, I didn't mind it so much."

If you think that "drugged" feeling is unpleasant, you can try taking cyclics right before bedtime or ask your doctor about lowering your dosage. Or you may have more luck with one of the nonsedating tricyclics: amoxapine, desipramine, nortriptyline, or protriptyline. These are a good choice if you experience lethargy and tiredness in addition to your depression. On the other hand, they may interfere with sleep, especially if you take your medication late in the day.

Neuroleptic Malignant Syndrome. If you use amoxapine too long, you run the small risk of developing a group of symptoms called "neuroleptic malignant syndrome," including fever, fast or irregular heartbeat, sweating, weakness, muscle stiffness, seizures, or loss of bladder control.

Sexual Problems. Most antidepressants affect sexual functioning in one way or another, and cyclics aren't any different. You may experience either an increase or a decrease in sexual interest. Men may experience problems with erection or ejaculation or suffer from impotence. Cyclics may trigger swollen testicles or breast enlargement in men and women. If you experience significant problems with sexual functioning, your doctor may choose to switch you to a different antidepressant that doesn't cause these problems, such as Wellbutrin (bupropion).

Sun Sensitivity. If you take a cyclic antidepressant and you go out into the sun even briefly, you may end up with a rash, red or discolored skin, or a dreadful sunburn. Before going out into the sun, study the accompanying list of "Sunlight Precautions When Taking Cyclic Antidepressants" (see box). If you do get a severe reaction from the sun, consult your doctor.

SUNLIGHT PRECAUTIONS
WHEN TAKING CYCLIC ANTIDEPRESSANTS

To prevent harmful skin reactions following exposure to sunlight, take the following precautions when you are taking cyclics:

➤ Stay out of direct sunlight between 10 A.M. and 3 P.M.
➤ If you have average skin, apply sunblock with an SPF of at least 15; for fair or extremely sensitive skin, use a higher SPF number.
➤ Apply a lip sunblock with an SPF of at least 15.
➤ Wear protective clothing, a scarf or hat, and sunglasses.
➤ Do not use tanning booths or beds or sunlamps.

Sweating. Doxepin may interfere with sweating, making it harder for your body to withstand heat. To avoid the risk of heat stroke, avoid saunas or extremely hot climates while taking this drug.

Tardive Dyskinesia. Amoxapine carries the risk of a group of unique side effects called "tardive dyskinesia"— speech or swallowing problems, lip smacking or puckering, loss of balance, cheek puffing, rapid or wormlike tongue movements, shakiness or trembling, shuffling walk, slow movements, arm or leg stiffness, uncontrolled chewing movements, and uncontrolled movements of hands, arms, or legs. This tardive dyskinesia may be permanent.

Weight Gain. Many of the tricyclics cause weight gain. While it begins with just a few pounds, long-term treatment can add more and more weight until people stop taking the antidepressant (one study found that 48 percent of people stopped taking tricyclics because of weight gain). While there aren't any specific restrictions on diet, you may want to guard against eating too much to avoid gaining too much weight. You can take clomipramine with meals or after eating to lessen stomach distress.

    If you're having a serious problem with weight gain, your doctor may want to consider one of the newer antidepressants (such as Wellbutrin, Paxil, Prozac, Zoloft, Desyrel, or Effexor), which don't usually cause weight gain.

Drug Interactions

Some medicines should never be used with cyclics (see box on pages 158 to 159, "Potential Drug Interactions with Cyclic Antidepressants"), but other drug combinations are okay as long as your doctor monitors your condition closely.

Of course you'll want to avoid alcohol, which can be toxic when combined with cyclics. Taking cocaine with cyclics may cause irregular heartbeat; smoking marijuana may make you too sleepy. Some experts also believe that tobacco may make cyclics less effective.

There are also some specific interactions with a few of the cyclics. If you're taking desipramine, you should know that the effects of estrogen or birth-control pills may decrease the antidepressant's effectiveness.

Lithium will decrease the effectiveness of imipramine; imipramine's effects will be strengthened by simultaneously taking Prozac, estrogens, Ritalin, or birth-control pills. In addition, this drug may mask poisoning by organophosphorous-type insecticides.

Ludiomil may increase the effect of anticoagulants and may decrease the effect of guanethidine. Increased sedation may result by combining Ludiomil and anti-cholinergics or central-nervous-system depressants. The affects of Ludiomil may be increased if taken with cimetidine, thiazide, or Prozac, and may be decreased if taken with clonidine. Toxic symptoms may follow a combination of Ludiomil with methylphenidate. Finally, Ludiomil combined with levodopa may increase blood pressure.

POTENTIAL DRUG INTERACTIONS
WITH CYCLIC ANTIDEPRESSANTS

➤ Alcohol
➤ Amphetamines (dextroamphetamine, methamphetamine)
➤ Anesthetics (plus some dental anesthetics)
➤ Aldomet
➤ Anticonvulsants (diazepam, phenobarbital, phenytoin, valproic acid, etc.)
➤ Antihistamines (Actifed, Benadryl, Chlor-Trimeton, Compoz, Dimetapp-DM)
➤ Appetite suppressants (fenfluramine, Preludin, Trimcaps, etc.)
➤ Barbiturates (Amytal, Nembutal, phenobarbital, Seconal, talbutal, etc.)
➤ Benzodiazepines (Dalmane, diazepam, Halcion, Librium, Valium, Xanax, etc.)
➤ Blood thinners (Coumadin, dicumarol, warfarin, etc.)
➤ Catapres
➤ Cylert
➤ Ephedrine (Broncholate, Ephed II, etc.)
➤ Hylorel
➤ Ismelin
➤ Isuprel
➤ MAOIs
➤ Muscle relaxants (cyclobenzaprine, dantrolene, orphenadrine, etc.)
➤ Neo-Synephrine
➤ Orap
➤ Phenergan
➤ Serpasil
➤ Sinus medications (Sinutab, Advil Sinus, etc.)

POTENTIAL DRUG INTERACTIONS
WITH CYCLIC ANTIDEPRESSANTS *(continued)*

➤ Tagamet
➤ Temaril
➤ Tranquilizers (buspirone, chlorpromazine, haloperidol, thiothixene, etc.)
➤ Wellbutrin

The effects of clomipramine may be increased if taken with Prozac, Haldol, some diuretics, and Tagamet. If taken with Dilantin, chloral hydrate, or lithium, its effects may be decreased.

The effects of desipramine may be increased if taken with phenothiazine and decreased if taken with chloral hydrate, estrogen, lithium, or birth-control pills.

Imipramine's effects may be increased by taking it simultaneously with Tagamet, Prozac, or Ritalin. Its effects may be decreased by taking chloral hydrate or lithium at the same time.

Nortriptyline increases the effects of dicumarol and the drug's effects may be increased if taken with Tagamet or quinidine.

Pregnancy and Breast-feeding

If you're pregnant and seriously depressed, you and your doctor will have to weigh the risks of your untreated depression against possible damage to your fetus.

Theoretically, all cyclics can pass into breast milk; therefore, you may want to discuss the wisdom of breast-feeding with your doctor if you are going to take cyclics after giving birth. The only specific negative information about tricyclics and breast-feeding infants is that doxepine may cause drowsiness in nursing babies.

Cyclics and Children

Imipramine is the most widely studied antidepressant when it comes to treating children. Because it's also one of the least toxic, it's the antidepressant most likely to be prescribed for youngsters. When a child is taking imipramine, his blood pressure, pulse, and heart rhythm should be monitored, since there's a greater risk of heart problems in youngsters between 6 and 12 than there is in adults. Despite extensive studies with children, no one knows whether this drug is safe for youngsters under age 6.

Imipramine is usually started at low doses (usually 25 milligrams daily) and increased by increments of 25 milligrams every few days until the depression begins to fade. Doses should always be given by an adult, since overdoses in children have been reported. Overdoses of tricyclics are particularly serious in children, who are unusually sensitive to these drugs. Doses should not exceed 2.5 milligrams per kilogram per day in children.

Because children are especially sensitive to all cyclics, they are at greater risk for side effects, especially nervousness, sleeping problems, fatigue, and mild stomach irritation. Check with your doctor if your child has any of these symptoms.

Cyclics and the Elderly

If you're over age 60 and take cyclics, don't be surprised if you experience one or more of these symptoms: confusion, dizziness, drowsiness, dry mouth, shakiness, fainting, constipation, urinary problems, headache, insomnia, and vision problems. Call your physician immediately if you experience any of these symptoms after you *stop* taking the drugs.

Cyclics and Obsessive-Compulsive Disorder

People with OCD become obsessed with certain thoughts and are bogged down with repetitive activities like washing themselves or rechecking doors and windows. The standard treatment for this disorder, which affects about 5 million Americans, is the tricyclic clomipramine, although in 1994 the FDA approved the SSRIs Prozac and Luvox as OCD treatments as well.

Because clomipramine must sometimes be taken in high doses (200 to 300 milligrams daily) to be effective against OCD, severe side effects are common. This is why more and more physicians are turning to SSRIs, which produce only very mild side effects with this group.

Withdrawal

Once you and your doctor decide it's time for you to stop taking cyclics, don't just throw out the bottle and go on your way. First of all, you'll need to be careful not to stop taking your medication too soon, because your depression might return with renewed force. And there could also be some unpleasant consequences to an abrupt withdrawal from these antidepressants.

Most doctors advise their patients to take cyclics from six months to a year for best results. Others take antidepressants for much longer without apparent ill effects.

"With my doctor's okay, I've cut down my dosage of imipramine from 350 milligrams a day to 150," reports Carol. "My doctor tells me it's up to me as to how I feel. Eventually, I hope I can stop altogether. But if I feel a problem coming on, I'll go back on imipramine to keep from being depressed." You'll need to slowly decrease the dose if you've taken a cyclic for a long time, in order to lessen the risk of headaches, nausea, and overall discomfort.

The specter of side effects won't disappear after you stop taking the drug, however. You need to be aware that with this particular group of antidepressants, there are some side effects that may crop up only *after* you stop taking them. Check with your doctor if you notice any of the following: headache, irritability, lip smacking or puckering, nausea or vomiting, diarrhea, abdominal pain, convulsions, puffing of cheeks, rapid wormlike tongue movements, restlessness, insomnia, vivid dreams, uncontrolled chewing movements, uncontrolled leg or arm movements, or unusual excitement.

And remember, the medicine's effects may last up to seven days after you've stopped taking the pills. Observe all precautions about drug interactions and sun exposure listed in this chapter until a week after your treatment has stopped.

Conclusion

This chapter has described the creation of the very first antidepressants—and how they're still being used successfully by many people today. The next chapter will continue the antidepressant evolution, introducing the monoamine oxidase inhibitors—MAOIs.

6

MONOAMINE OXIDASE INHIBITORS (MAOIs)

"MAO inhibitors worked much better for me than tricyclics. But for a chocoholic, the dietary restrictions were torture. That's why I finally stopped taking them."

—*Marie, 42*

Soon after scientists developed tricyclic antidepressants, another group of chemicals very different from the tricyclics rolled out of the laboratory—the monoamine oxidase (MAO) inhibitors. These new drugs affected the same neurotransmitters (serotonin and norepinephrine) that the tricyclics did, but they also affected dopamine.

How MAOIs Work

Once the brain's three neurotransmitters, known as monoamines (serotonin, norepinephrine, and dopamine), have played their part in sending messages in the brain, they get burned up by a protein in the brain called monoamine oxidase, a liver and brain enzyme.

Antidepressants known as monoamine oxidase inhibitors work by blocking this cleanup activity. When the excess neurotransmitters don't get destroyed, they start piling up in the brain. And since depression is associated with low levels of these monoamines, it's not surprising that *increasing* the monoamines ease depressive symptoms.

Unfortunately, monoamine oxidase doesn't just destroy those neurotransmitters; it's also responsible for mopping up another amine called tyramine, a molecule that affects blood pressure. So when monoamine oxidase gets blocked, levels of tyramine begin to rise, too. And that's when the trouble starts.

While a hike in neurotransmitters is beneficial, an increase in tyramine is disastrous. Excess tyramine can cause a sudden, sometimes fatal increase in blood pressure so severe that it can burst blood vessels in the brain.

Every time you eat chicken liver, aged cheese, broad-bean pods, or pickled herring, tyramine floods into

TYPES OF MAO INHIBITORS AND THEIR DOSAGES

MAOI	USUAL STARTING DOSE	MAXIMUM DOSE
phenelzine (Nardil)	15 mg/day	60 mg/day
tranylcypromine (Parnate)	30 mg/day	60 mg/day

your brain. Normally, MAO enzymes take care of this potentially harmful tyramine excess. But if you're taking an MAO inhibitor, the MAO enzyme can't stop tyramine from building up. This is exactly what happened when the drugs were introduced in the 1960s. Because no one knew about the tyramine connection, a wave of deaths from brain hemorrhages swept the country. Other patients taking MAO inhibitors experienced severe headaches caused by the rise in blood pressure. These early side effects were particularly disturbing because nobody knew why they were happening.

The mystery was solved when a British pharmacist noticed that his wife, who was taking MAO inhibitors, got headaches when she ate cheese. But the early MAOIs were considered so dangerous (they also can damage the liver, brain, and cardiovascular system) that even after the MAO-tyramine connection was finally understood, these drugs were taken off the American market for a time. (A related European antidepressant drug, Deprenyl, is marketed in this country as an anti-Parkinson's medication; it requires less stringent dietary cautions.)

Eventually the MAOIs were reintroduced in this country despite the tyramine risk because some depressed people don't respond to any other medication. Nevertheless, MAO inhibitors are usually the antidepressants of last resort.

"I call it the 'St. Jude' drug," says psychiatrist Andy Myerson. "It's the drug I use when nothing else works and someone is willing to give up anything in the hope that something will help their depression."

Prime Candidates

If you're very vulnerable to depression but don't suffer from the classic symptoms of major depression, MAOIs could be for you. They are especially good if you seem mildly depressed, if you become depressed more gradually, or if your primary complaints are boredom and apathy. If you have atypical depression—you're sensitive to rejection, overeat and oversleep, and react strongly to your environment—you may respond very well to MAOIs, which can reduce the sensitivity that causes you to feel so easily hurt or rejected. Others who tend to respond very well to MAOIs can feel quite depressed, but they're able to surface from the morass of their depression from time to time and experience pleasure before plunging into depression again.

The MAOI phenelzine (Nardil) has been found specifically to help patients characterized as atypical. These patients often have mixed anxiety and depression, or depression with phobia or hypochondriacal features. There is less evidence that Nardil may be effective in severely depressed patients. Tranylcypromine (Parnate) is a good choice if you have major depression without melancholia.

Who Shouldn't Take MAOIs

If you've got serious heart problems, epilepsy, bronchitis, asthma, or high blood pressure, or if you resist following a stringent diet, MAOIs aren't for you. Studies suggest that Nardil may not be as effective if you are severely depressed. Patients should wait at least two weeks when being transferred to Parnate from another MAO inhibitor.

Pros and Cons

One of the big problems with MAO inhibitors is that they may make you feel drugged and sluggish. "I didn't respond to tricyclics at all five years ago," says Karen, a New Jersey graduate student who has been chronically depressed most of her life. "When I was switched to an MAOI, I responded very well. But I couldn't take the diet. After I finally went off the drug, my friends told me I was always in a daze while I was taking MAOIs, but I wasn't aware of that at the time. I was switched to Prozac four years ago, and I've been taking that ever since." Patients often look dazed or even robotic, much the way Karen had appeared to her friends. But what people really hate are the lists of dietary restrictions and potential side effects.

"A lot of patients are resentful about the diet they have to follow," explains Dr. Myerson. "They tend to blame the doctor when they can't eat their favorite foods, and many people simply won't follow the diet." Other mental health experts point out that MAO inhibitors often interfere with the relationship between doctor and patient, because people feel so resentful about their side effects and diet that they don't want to talk to their doctor during therapy.

Their relatively risky profile makes them a poor choice for potentially suicidal patients who might intentionally take an overdose. At very low doses, the MAOIs can have toxic effects on the heart, unlike Prozac, which is not considered toxic even at very high doses. Studies have shown that MAOIs are not associated *at all* with suicide in nonsuicidal patients, as opposed to most other antidepressants. In a 1991 Harvard University study of 1,017 depressed people, 63 nonsuicidal patients took an MAOI and none became suicidal.

On the other hand, there's no doubt that for a certain subset of people, the MAO inhibitors work better than any other antidepressant.

"I've seen a few miracle cures with these drugs," one psychiatrist noted. "And they're particularly good if people suffer from panic attacks in addition to depression."

Furthermore, if you have hypertension or heart problems, the MAOIs might be for you because at therapeutic doses, they can *lower* blood pressure. In contrast to the tricyclic antidepressants, MAO inhibitors have little negative effect on heart rate.

If you were having problems with chest pain (angina) before taking MAO inhibitors, you may find that you're feeling much better now that you're taking this drug. Whatever you do, don't start running a few extra miles or working out a lot more at the gym without first discussing it with your doctor! Too much activity can bring on another attack of chest pain.

Before Taking MAOIs

Your doctor will probably quiz you about a range of medical conditions before prescribing an MAO inhibitor. *It's especially important to tell your doctor if you have frequent headaches or chest pain.* Since a severe headache or chest pain during MAOI therapy is the primary warning sign of a serious spike in blood pressure, anyone who *normally* gets severe headaches might overlook an important warning sign.

Your doctor will want to know if you have diabetes mellitus (you may need to change your insulin level) or an alcohol problem, since drinking while taking MAOIs may cause serious side effects.

Also tell your doctor if you have heart or blood-vessel disease, liver or kidney problems, Parkinson's disease, or an overactive thyroid.

Side Effects

The one thing you've got to watch out for with these drugs is that sudden spike in blood pressure called a "hypertensive crisis" (also called the "cheese reaction") that we discussed at the beginning of this chapter. As long as you follow a strict tyramine-free diet (see box on page 172, "Dietary Restrictions"), you should be able to avoid the risk.

Diet-Related Side Effects. Your doctor most assuredly will give you a list of prohibited foods. It's important to remember that the tyramine found in foods—even a type of food that can be eaten in small quantities—adds up. So while it's okay to eat small amounts of sour cream or arti-chokes, it would not be acceptable to eat a meal of sauer-kraut with a sauce of yogurt and sour cream, followed by a dessert of raspberries and chocolate together with a cup of coffee.

It's also important to understand that while you may get away with eating a forbidden food once or twice, it may cause a reaction the third or fourth time. This is because a particular food doesn't always contain the same amount of tyramine.

DIETARY RESTRICTIONS

Don't eat or drink any of the following when taking MAOIs unless your doctor advises otherwise:

➤ Aged foods
➤ Alcoholic beverages (especially Chianti, sherry, and liqueurs)
➤ Alcohol-free or reduced-alcohol beer or wine
➤ Anchovies
➤ Bologna, pepperoni, salami, summer sausage, or any fermented sausage
➤ Caviar
➤ Cheeses (especially strong or aged varieties), except for cottage and cream cheese
➤ Chicken livers
➤ Fermented foods
➤ Figs (canned)
➤ Fruit—raisins, bananas (or any overripe fruit)
➤ Meat prepared with tenderizers; unfresh meat; meat extracts
➤ Smoked or pickled meat, poultry, or fish
➤ Soy sauce

Foods you can eat in moderation:
➤ Avocados
➤ Beer
➤ Caffeine (including chocolate, coffee, tea, cola)
➤ Chocolate
➤ Raspberries
➤ Sauerkraut
➤ Soup (canned or powdered)
➤ Sour cream
➤ Yogurt

The symptoms are as follows: severe headache radiating to the front of the head, stiff and/or sore neck, nausea and vomiting, sensitivity to light, dilated pupils, sweating (sometimes with fever or with cold, clammy skin), chest pain, or heart palpitations. A blood pressure rise usually occurs within several hours after taking the drug. *Stop taking MAO inhibitors immediately if you get a severe headache or palpitations,* then call your doctor.

Your doctor can give you a drug called Procardia as an emergency measure if you accidentally eat something that causes a reaction.

There is also a range of less serious side effects that accompany the MAOIs. Like all antidepressants, the MAOIs are capable of inducing a manic state in people who are manic-depressive. Like tricyclics, MAOIs have been reported to cause memory problems. Other possible side effects follow.

Fainting and/or Dizziness. If you're taking an MAOI, you may feel a bit dizzy or faint if you stand up quickly. It's a common side effect with these drugs and it is more annoying than anything else. It can lead to giddiness, muscular weakness, nausea, perspiration, hyperventilation, and sometimes confusion. If this happens to you, try standing up more slowly. (You may notice that you have a particular problem when you get up in the morning; this is because blood pressure is lowest then. If this happens, sit on the edge of the bed, dangling your feet for a minute or two, and then rise slowly.)

This problem often fades away with time. If it doesn't, you can try exercising your leg muscles to prevent blood

GENERAL SIDE EFFECTS OF ALL MAO INHIBITORS

Stop taking this drug and seek immediate help for:
- Unusually high blood pressure
- Fast or slow heartbeat
- Severe headache
- Increased sweating
- Increased sensitivity to light
- Severe chest pain
- Stiff or sore neck
- Nausea and vomiting

Check with your doctor if you have:
- Severe dizziness or lightheadedness, especially when arising from a sitting or lying position
- Pounding heartbeat
- Fever
- Slurred speech
- Staggering walk
- Diarrhea
- Swelling of feet and/or lower legs
- Unusual excitement or nervousness
- Dark urine
- Skin rash
- Sore throat
- Yellow eyes and/or skin

Mild side effects not usually requiring medical attention:
- Blurry vision
- Urinary problems
- Mild headache
- Increased sweating
- Shakiness or trembling
- Sleeping problems
- Constipation
- Dry mouth
- Increased appetite (especially for sweets)
- Mild dizziness or lightheadedness
- Decreased sexual ability
- Drowsiness
- Weight gain
- Restlessness
- Fatigue and weakness
- Chills
- Decreased appetite
- Muscle twitching during sleep

from pooling in your legs. It may also help to wear support hosiery and drink plenty of fluids.

If the problem gets worse, ask your doctor if you can divide your medication into several doses to be taken during the day. Try taking the medicine after meals, and take salt tablets.

Drowsiness. Because MAO inhibitors may cause blurred vision, drowsiness, or a "drugged" feeling, be sure you know how you react to this medicine before you do anything that could be dangerous if your alertness or vision were affected, such as driving or operating machinery.

Diabetes. If you're a diabetic, MAO inhibitors may affect your blood sugar levels. While using these antidepressants, be very careful when you're testing the sugar levels in your blood or urine. Consult with your doctor if you have any questions about your diabetic condition.

Sexual Problems. Like many other antidepressants, MAOIs can cause a range of sexual problems. Of these, delayed orgasm is the most common (it is also very likely with Prozac). However, many people note that sexual problems eventually disappear.

Surgery. Be sure to tell your doctor or dentist that you're taking MAO inhibitors before any kind of surgery, dental treatment, or emergency treatment—even if you stopped taking the drug up to two weeks ago. The anesthesia combined with the MAOIs can cause a drop in blood pressure or other problems. You may want to carry an ID card noting that you're taking this medicine. If you're taking these drugs, you shouldn't agree to any elective surgery requiring general anesthesia.

Weight Gain. MAOIs are associated with some degree of weight gain. (Prozac and some other SSRIs do not seem to cause this side effect.)

Drug Interactions

While aspirin, Tylenol (plain), Motrin, or antibiotics are safe when combined with MAOIs, you should check with your doctor before taking *any other medicine.*

There have been reports of serious—sometimes fatal—reactions when an MAO inhibitor is combined with SSRIs. These reactions include high blood pressure, nausea and vomiting, fever, rigidity, rapidly fluctuating vital signs, shock, and mental changes. You shouldn't take an SSRI until two weeks after stopping therapy with an MAO inhibitor. Even more important, because these drugs take a long time to be eliminated from the body, *you should wait at least five weeks after stopping an SSRI before you start taking an MAO inhibitor.*

Besides SSRIs, there are some other medications that can provoke a hypertensive reaction similar to the cheese reaction (but not involving tyramine). Of these, the most dangerous are nonprescription cold, cough, or sinus medications such as Contac or Dristan; most of them contain decongestants (like pseudoephedrine). Other drugs on the danger list include weight-control pills and asthma inhalants. Illegal drugs like cocaine and amphetamines also cause this problem.

Most of the medications that cause problems are stimulants that can trigger an increase in the release of norepinephrine, which raises blood pressure. Since MAO metabolizes norepinephrine, people taking MAOIs have higher amounts of norepinephrine to be released, which raises the blood level of norepinephrine even more.

The opiate narcotics Demerol (meperidine) and dextromethorphan (found in cough or cold medicines usually labeled "DM") should also be avoided. And Parnate can interfere with the benefit of guanethidine, methyldopa, reserpine, and dopamine. Nardil shouldn't be taken with dopamine, epinephrine and norepinephrine, methyldopa, L-dopa, L-tryptophan, L-tyrosine, or phenylalanine (contained in aspartame, also known as NutraSweet).

Overdose

The MAO inhibitors are somewhat more dangerous drugs than other antidepressants when taken in excessive amounts—far more so than the SSRIs. Symptoms of overdose include severe anxiety, confusion, convulsions or seizures, cool clammy skin, severe dizziness, severe drowsiness, fast and irregular pulse, fever, hallucinations, severe headache, high or low blood pressure, muscle stiffness, breathing problems, severe sleeping problems, or unusual irritability.

Tolerance

Some people develop a tolerance to MAO inhibitors. This could mean that the drug will work for you at first, but you could suddenly become depressed again in the middle

DRUG INTERACTIONS AND MAO INHIBITORS

Some drugs should never be combined with MAO inhibitors, while others may be used if your doctor adjusts your dosage. It's extremely important for you to tell your doctor if you are taking any of the following drugs:

➤ Allergy medicines (including nose drops or sprays)
➤ Appetite suppressants
➤ Antihistamines (Actifed DM, Benadryl, Benylin, Chlor-Trimeton, Compoz, etc.)
➤ Antipsychotics
➤ Antivert
➤ Asthma drugs
➤ Atrovent
➤ Blood-pressure medicine
➤ Bucladin
➤ BuSpar (may cause high blood pressure)
➤ Cocaine (may severely increase blood pressure)
➤ Cold medicines
➤ Demerol (deaths have occurred when combining MAOIs and a single dose of meperidine)
➤ Dextromethorphan (may cause brief episodes of psychosis or bizarre behavior)
➤ Ditropan
➤ Dopar, Larodopa
➤ Flexeril
➤ Insulin (MAOIs may change amount of insulin needed)
➤ Ludiomil
➤ Marezine
➤ Monoamine oxidase inhibitors (other)

DRUG INTERACTIONS AND MAO INHIBITORS
(continued)

➤ Norflex
➤ Norpace
➤ Phenergan
➤ Pronestyl
➤ Prozac (may cause high fever, rigidity, high blood pressure, mental changes, confusion and hypomania; at least five weeks should pass between stopping Prozac and starting an MAOI)
➤ Quinidex
➤ Ritalin
➤ Sinus medicine
➤ Symmetrel
➤ Tegretol (may increase seizures)
➤ Temaril (may increase chance of side effects)
➤ Tricyclic antidepressants (using these drugs within two weeks of taking MAOIs may cause serious side effects including sudden fever, extremely high blood pressure, convulsions, and death)
➤ Tryptophan (may cause disorientation, confusion, amnesia, delirium, agitation, hypomanic signs, shivering)
➤ Urispas
➤ Wellbutrin (allow at least two weeks between stopping Wellbutrin and starting MAOIs)

of treatment. This sort of reaction is particularly disturbing because it sets off a plummeting depression that may not respond to any other antidepressant. Oddly, if you develop tolerance to an MAOI, the best solution may be to switch to another antidepressant for a few weeks, and then start taking the same MAOI again. This way, the drug may regain its effectiveness.

Withdrawal

Don't suddenly stop taking this medicine on your own. Your doctor will probably ask you to gradually taper off your dosage to avoid the risk of side effects. Once you do stop taking the drug, remember that you must continue to observe all the dietary restrictions *for at least two weeks*, avoiding all the same foods and beverages that you did when you were taking MAO inhibitors.

Pregnancy and Breast-feeding

Because Parnate (and most likely Nardil) cross the placenta, you and your doctor should weigh the need for this drug against the risks to your unborn child. Nardil has been shown to have adverse effects in pregnant mice; in doses well above the human dose it has caused decreases in the number of healthy offspring. While researchers don't know for sure whether anti-depressants cause birth defects in humans, women who take any type of antidepressant have about twice the rate of miscarriages during the first trimester of pregnancy. As with most antidepressants, safe use of MAO inhibitors during pregnancy hasn't been established, but one limited study in humans did suggest an increased risk of birth defects when MAOIs are taken during the first trimester.

In animals, MAO inhibitors slow the growth of newborns and make them more excitable when their mothers take very large doses during pregnancy.

When it comes to breast-feeding, Parnate is passed into breast milk, but it is not known if this is true of Nardil. There haven't been any reports of problems in nursing infants whose mothers have taken MAO inhibitors.

MAOIs and Children

Because MAOIs are among the most risky of the antidepressants, most experts don't recommend giving them to children under age 16. Animal studies indicate that these drugs may slow growth in the young.

MAOIs and the Elderly

Older patients are usually more sensitive than younger adults to the MAO inhibitors, and they may be more likely to experience dizziness or lightheadedness. Because of the danger of an abrupt increase in high blood pressure (hypertensive crisis), the MAO inhibitors are often not prescribed for people over age 60, or for those with heart or blood-vessel diseases.

Parnate should not be routinely given to anyone over age 60 because of the possibility of damaged blood vessels and the risk of sudden high blood pressure; you should wait at least two weeks before being transferred from Parnate to another MAOI. In this event, the starting dose should be half the normal starting dose for the first week of therapy.

Other Uses

MAOIs have been shown to be effective in the treatment of a wide range of disorders besides depression. They are very good at treating eating disorders—but the weight gain they often cause can be counterproductive. Prozac, on the other hand, is just as effective as an eating-disorder treatment, without the unwanted side effects. In one recent study of 400 women, Prozac cut down on eating binges in 63 percent of the responders and vomiting in up to 57 percent.

For social phobics, for whom the idea of a social occasion can produce a range of negative emotions and symptoms, MAOIs (especially Nardil) can be very helpful. In fact, studies suggest that about 70 percent of people who are social phobics respond to MAOIs. Recent research has suggested that Prozac may also be effective for this problem.

MAOIs are also helpful in treating panic disorder, social phobia, agoraphobia, obsessive-compulsive disorder, and attention-deficit disorder.

Conclusion

You've seen how difficult the MAOIs can be, and how helpful they are to a subgroup of people who respond well to them. In the next chapter, we'll learn about drugs used to treat bipolar disorder (manic-depression): Zyprexa, lithium, Tegretol, Depakote, anticonvulsants, and benzodiazepines.

7 BIPOLAR DISORDER (MANIC-DEPRESSION)

"When I went off lithium, the manic-depression came back. I was barely able to go to work. It was terrible. I would stand there at work and pretend I was alive."

—Jack, 48

Jack had been consumed with energy all his life, but in his early twenties he experienced his first heavy depression. Diagnosed with a classic case of bipolar disorder (manic-depression), he began taking lithium and was able to live a fairly normal life until 1989, when his doctors briefly stopped his lithium treatment.

During this period, Jack spiraled into a state he describes as "close to death," a depression so profound he didn't know whether he would survive. By the time he was put back on lithium, he no longer responded to the drug. Now considered to be "lithium resistant," he takes a combination of the antiepileptics Tegretol and Depakote.

For Jack, the combination "is only about 40 percent effective," he says. Jack is a "rapid cycler," with a mixed state of manic-depression. This means that instead of extended episodes of depression and then mania lasting for several months each, he cycles constantly through mania and depression. The drugs he takes don't eradicate this process, but they tone it down so that his lows aren't quite so devastating and his highs aren't quite so manic.

Lithium

Lithium is an element of the periodic table that readily forms salts. As early as 200 A.D., the Greek physician Galen was prescribing alkaline spring baths for manic patients.

Lithium *bromide* was used as a sedative beginning in the early 1900s, but it fell into disfavor in the 1940s when some heart patients died after using it as a salt substitute. Almost immediately thereafter, a little-known psychiatrist in Australia discovered that lithium salts were extremely effective in treating manic-depression.

Eventually, lithium's popularity grew, until by the late 1960s it was once again widely prescribed in this country, when it was heralded as the first effective treatment for manic-depression.

Excreted by the kidneys, lithium *carbonate* has a narrow range between toxic and therapeutic doses. It's used mostly to manage manic-depression, to smooth out the hills and valleys of a person's emotional swings and the lows of chronic recurring depression. It can quickly reverse acute mania in 80 percent of people, and stabilize mood in 60 to 70 percent.

How Does It Work?

While scientists aren't quite sure how this drug works, they believe it may correct chemical imbalances in certain nerve impulse transmitters (serotonin and norepinephrine) that influence emotional status and behavior.

While lithium can have a mild antidepressant effect, it's primarily effective for its strong anti-manic effects, working best by controlling the highs of mania. If you're taking lithium to control manic highs but you're still depressed, your doctor may want to add Prozac or another antidepressant, which is helpful for long-term control of manic-depression.

Lithium can also be effective in the treatment of major depression, and can boost the effectiveness of tricyclics, MAOIs, or SSRIs when these drugs don't quite get the job done on their own.

Is Lithium for Everyone?

Unfortunately, lithium doesn't work well for everyone. About 20 percent of people will have a complete remission on lithium, and the rest will have varying degrees of relief. Some will experience fewer episodes of mania; those episodes that do occur are shorter and less severe, and people feel more stable between manic episodes. But for some people, lithium may just stop working.

Lithium no longer works for Jack, whose partially uncontrolled manic-depression is so debilitating he can't work. In his depressed state, he can't concentrate, can't read, feels lethargic, and has memory problems. Then he'll suddenly shoot up into mania, with too much energy and a "horrible libido."

Jack's case is an example of a person with progressive manic-depression, whose disorder worsens over time; lithium can stop working for these people, and the alternatives (Tegretol and Depakote) may not be completely effective. Because some experts believe that progressive manic-depression is a result of structural changes in the brain as the disease worsens, they recommend keeping people on lithium for long periods of time to prevent the almost-impossible-to-reverse deterioration. (This theory is controversial.)

In about 30 percent of manic-depressives, lithium smooths out the periods of mania but it doesn't control the episodes of depression. If this is your problem, your doctor may combine Prozac (or another SSRI) with lithium. On the other hand, you shouldn't take Prozac without lithium if you have bipolar I manic-depression, since Prozac could push you into an out-of-control manic high. (Bipolar I is a severe form of manic-depression characterized by dark periods of deep depression alternating with highs so manic a person may require hospitalization.)

Who Shouldn't Take Lithium

You shouldn't take lithium if you have uncontrolled diabetes or untreated hypoglycemia (low blood sugar), or if you can't have your blood levels regularly tested. Nursing mothers and those allergic to lithium shouldn't take this medication either.

Who Benefits from Lithium

While the standard patient who takes lithium is diagnosed as a manic-depressive, it may also be given in combination with other antidepressants to a depressed person with a familial history of manic-depression.

"My doctor wanted me to go on lithium because my brother is manic-depressive," says Eleanor, 38. "I didn't want to take it, because my brother takes lithium and he's really sick. I had an aversion to being diagnosed manic-depressive."

In fact, lithium alone did *not* help Eleanor, but when her psychiatrist combined it with the SSRI Paxil, her depression began to respond. "My psychiatrist says that Paxil helped my depression, and the lithium helped keep me from getting manic," she says. "I take 450 milligrams of lithium twice a day, and Paxil in the afternoon. I feel lighter. People started saying I look younger."

How to Take Lithium

Lithium will only work when it reaches the correct level in the bloodstream. The effective level of lithium is about the same for everybody. However, you can't just pop a pill and assume that the lithium level is correct. Regular blood tests are necessary to make sure that the correct level of the drug is maintained. These tests are not only critical in determining whether the patient is getting enough lithium, but they also guard against getting too much. This is important because the level needed to correct mania and depression is very close to a level that can make you sick (see box on page 188, "Lithium Toxicity Symptoms").

Before you're given lithium, your doctor will arrange for an EKG, blood tests, and urine tests. Periodically, these tests will need to be repeated as part of your monitoring. To guard against lithium toxicity,

---

LITHIUM TOXICITY SYMPTOMS

Remember: It's easy for toxic levels of lithium to build up if you have kidney problems or low salt levels, if you get dehydrated or take diuretics, or during childbirth.

EARLY SIGNS
- Diarrhea and vomiting
- Drowsiness
- Muscular weakness
- Lack of coordination

HIGHER TOXICITY
- Giddiness/confusion
- Blurred vision
- Tinnitus (ringing of the ears)
- Seizures
- Staggering gait

---

your doctor will need to measure the level of lithium in your blood to make sure you're not getting too much. This may seem inconvenient, but remember that inadequate monitoring can have fatal results. In the beginning, your doctor will probably monitor your blood level once a week until your dosage is stabilized, drawing blood levels 10 to 12 hours after your last dose. Once you're stabilized and taking maintenance therapy, your blood levels should be checked in a month, and then every three months.

To lessen the chance of stomach irritation, it's a good idea to take lithium with or after meals. It usually takes from one to three weeks to notice an improvement in your mania and several months to ease the depression.

Patients experiencing acute mania are usually started out with at least 900 milligrams of lithium carbonate per day, although dosage is regulated according to blood levels and response.

Dietary Restrictions

While you're taking lithium, you should never restrict your use of salt; too little could increase lithium's effect. Don't drink too much tea and coffee, which increases the risk of adverse effects. Drink plenty of liquids (at least 8 to 12 glasses of water each day), and don't skip meals. Don't drink alcohol at all with lithium.

Side Effects

More common and less dangerous side effects may include thirst and frequent urination (see box on page 190, "Side Effects of Lithium"). Some people also gain weight during the first few months that they take lithium. A sensitivity to lithium might make you drowsy.

You should contact your doctor at the *first* sign of toxicity: drowsiness, sluggishness, unsteadiness, tremor, muscle twitching, vomiting, or diarrhea. If you have a mild case of toxicity, your doctor will probably just discontinue lithium temporarily, and give you fluids and electrolytes. Because more severe cases can cause lasting brain damage or death, serious lithium poisoning usually requires aggressive treatment with hemodialysis.

If you have psoriasis or diabetes, you may notice your disease worsens during treatment with lithium.

Because it's important not to lose too much salt while you take lithium, be careful not to sweat too

SIDE EFFECTS OF LITHIUM

COMMON

➤ Anorexia ➤ Shakiness
➤ Diarrhea ➤ Thirst
➤ Dizziness ➤ Tremor
➤ Mouth dryness ➤ Frequent urination
➤ Sexual problems ➤ Vomiting

INFREQUENT

➤ Acne ➤ Weight gain
➤ Ear noises ➤ Shortness of breath
➤ Fainting ➤ Speech slurring
➤ Fatigue ➤ Stomach pain
➤ Muscle aches ➤ Headache
➤ Swelling ➤ Menstrual problems
➤ Rash (hands ➤ Heartbeat
and feet) irregularities
➤ Thyroid problems
(coldness; dry,
puffy skin)

RARE

➤ Hair loss ➤ Psoriasis worsening
➤ Eye pain ➤ Blurry vision
➤ Arm and/or
leg jerks

much, which can deplete body stores of salt and water and cause lithium toxicity. Avoid extremely hot climates and sauna baths for the same reason, and be careful of any illness that causes fever, sweating, vomiting, or diarrhea. This can also significantly alter the blood-lithium concentration, so you'll need to monitor blood levels if you get sick.

If you're over age 60, you may have more frequent or severe side effects than do younger people. Lithium isn't usually given to anyone under age 12.

Drug Interactions

It appears that while some people are good candidates for a lithium-SSRI combination, others aren't. While several reports have found that SSRIs can interfere with lithium, the two drugs used together can help some depressed people who don't respond to either drug alone.

When taking lithium, you shouldn't take over-the-counter medications that contain iodide (such as some cough medicines and vitamin-mineral supplements), because these drugs may affect the thyroid when taken with lithium.

Use caution if you combine lithium with Tegretol, chlorpromazine (Thorazine), phenothiazines, SSRIs, Haldol, or methyldopa (Aldomet). In addition, lithium may increase the effects of tricyclic antidepressants.

The effects of lithium may be increased if you take Bumex, Edecrin, Prozac, furosemide (Lasix), Indocin, Feldene, or some diuretics. Some other drugs may decrease the effects of lithium, including acetazolamide (Diamox), sodium bicarbonate, or theophylline (Theo-Dur).

There may be an increased risk of seizures by combining lithium with bupropion (Wellbutrin). Some drugs can also interact with lithium to produce toxicity, including some nonsteroidal anti-inflammatory drugs (such as ibuprofen).

Using cocaine or marijuana while taking lithium could cause psychosis.

Children and the Elderly

A safe effective level of lithium, as with many other anti-depressants, hasn't been established for children under 12. If you're over age 60, you may need to take smaller-than-standard doses, beginning with a test dose of 75 to 150 milligrams daily. Be especially careful when taking lithium if you're on a low-salt diet and you use diuretics.

Pregnancy and Breast-feeding

Lithium therapy throughout the first trimester of pregnancy and beyond may be associated with birth defects (especially the heart). Studies have also shown that if the baby's blood level of lithium reaches toxic levels before birth, the child may have "floppy infant" syndrome (weakness, lethargy, unresponsiveness, low temperature, a weak cry, and poor appetite). Rat and mice pups exposed to lithium before birth have been born with defects of the ear, eye, and palate. *You should stop taking lithium immediately if you're trying to get pregnant, or if you've just conceived.*

Because lithium is found in breast milk in significant amounts, doctors also recommend that you not plan to nurse if you use lithium.

Withdrawal

Suddenly stopping lithium medication doesn't cause any withdrawal symptoms. However, it's not a good idea to stop taking lithium too soon, since this may cause a return of either mania or depression. Some people may need treatment for at least a year. Don't stop taking lithium without talking to your doctor.

Long-Term Effects

Some people on long-term maintenance may experience altered thyroid function or goiter. Patients with kidney problems before starting on lithium often run into further kidney problems after using lithium for some time. (If you have kidney problems, you could either switch to Tegretol or Depakote.)

For some people with major depressive disorder and no history of mania or hypomania, Depakote alone can be very helpful in easing symptoms. In one recent study of three outpatients at the Dallas VA Mental Health Clinic, two-thirds of depressed patients responded well to the drug.

Your doctor may ask for follow-up medical exams or lab studies, such as an electrocardiogram, thyroid- or kidney-function tests, or complete blood counts.

Other Drug Choices

In the past few years, there have been dramatic changes in the treatment of bipolar disorder. Zyprexa, a new anti-psychotic drug, has been approved for mania. Second generation mood-stabilizing anticonvulsants Tegretol and Depakote are now widely used as alternatives to lithium or in combination with the "old standard." High-potency benzodiazepines are also used today as alternatives. In addition, third generation mood-stabilizing anticonvulsants have been used successfully to treat resistant bipolar disorder, including lamotrigine (Lamictal) and topiramate (Topamax). These two are approved by the FDA as anti-convulsants, but they are also used by doctors to regulate mood as an off label indication.

Zyprexa

The newest drug to be approved is the schizophrenia drug Zyprexa (olanzapine), which was approved in March 2000 by the FDA for the short-term treatment of acute manic episodes associated with bipolar disorder. Research suggests it provides better control of symptoms than Depakote.

Mania is the period of abnormal elation and irritability often accompanied by an unrealistic belief in one's own abilities. There may be increases in sex drive, delusions, and substance abuse. Depression may appear at the same time, or the person may cycle from mania to depression and back again.

Studies suggest that Zyprexa stabilizes mood to help manage the manic phase of bipolar disorder. Unlike some other drugs, it doesn't require blood monitoring. Since most patients with bipolar disorder seek treatment during depression, their mania may go undiagnosed at first.

Zyprexa caused a few side effects; those that were reported included dry mouth, drowsiness, dizziness, and loss of strength. However, the FDA cautions that life-threatening pancreatitis has occurred in some adults and children.

The beginning dose of Zyprexa to treat mania is 10 to 15 milligrams once a day at any time, without regard to meals. Used in the United States to treat psychotic disorders such as schizophrenia since 1996, it has been used by nearly 4 million people worldwide.

Lamotrigine and Topiramate

Lamotrigine and topiramate seem to be effective in about two-thirds of those patients who haven't responded to antidepressants or mood stabilizers without serious side effects. Both drugs can control rapid cycling and mixed bipolar states in those who haven't been helped by either Tegretol or Depakote. Further, some people who haven't been able to take antidepressants because the drugs triggered mania or agitation find that they can tolerate antidepressants when taking lamotrigine or topiramate at the same time. Both drugs are better at controlling depression than Tegretol or Depakote.

Before taking these drugs, you need a thorough medical examination with blood and urine tests to rule out any medical problem.

Dosage

While some patients notice an effect right away, it may take up to a month before any of these medications affect symptoms.

For lamotrigine, the initial dose is 25 milligrams once or twice daily, increased by 25 or 50 milligrams each week. Patients also taking Depakote are usually started on 12.5 milligrams a day, increased by 12.5 or 25 milligrams every two weeks. Those also taking Tegretol may be given somewhat larger doses of lamotrigine and more rapid dosage increases.

For topiramate, the first dose is usually between 12.5 and 25 milligrams a day, up to an eventual final dose of 100 to 200 milligrams per day (although some people need as much as 400 milligrams per day, especially when this drug is used alone).

Interactions with Depakote and Tegretol

No significant harmful interactions have been reported between these drugs and lithium, Depakote, or Tegretol. However, combining topiramate and lamotrigine with Depakote or Tegretol may alter the concentrations of the drugs in the body.

When taken with topiramate, Depakote or Tegretol can lower the concentration of topiramate in the bloodstream. Topiramate has no effect on the blood levels of Tegretol, but it can lower the concentration of Depakote.

Patients taking Tegretol and lamotrigine together may have slightly lower blood levels of lamotrigine; and Depakote can double the blood levels of lamotrigine.

Drug Interactions

Unlike many other antidepressants, these drugs may be used at the same time as an MAOI without problems. Only a few drug interactions have been reported.

➤ *Phenytoin (Dilantin):* lowers the concentration of topiramate in the body by 50 percent

➤ *Alcohol:* may worsen side effects in topiramate or lamotrigine

➤ *Phenobarbital:* lowers the blood level of lamotrigine by 40 percent

➤ *Primidone:* lowers the blood level of lamotrigine by 40 percent

Side Effects

The drugs do have different patterns of side effects. The most potentially serious side effect is with the drug lamotrigine, which may cause a rash ranging in severity from mild sunburn to a sometimes fatal condition in 1 out of 1,000 adults (the incidence in children is much higher). If you are taking this drug, report *all* rashes to your doctor. A rash is more likely to develop if you take high doses right away or if the drug is started too quickly when you are taking Depakote. Rarely, lamotrigine causes agitation, anxiety, concentration problems, confusion, irritability, and mania.

Topiramate may cause psychomotor slowing (4.1 percent), memory problems (3.3 percent), fatigue (3.3 percent), confusion (3.2 percent), and sleepiness (3.2 percent). In rare cases, it may cause sedation, anxiety, and confusion. Olanzapine has caused somnolence, dry mouth, dizziness, and weight gain.

Pregnancy and Breast-feeding

These drugs are listed as pregnancy category C, which means that animal studies have shown harmful effects on the fetus; but there are no adequate human studies. The benefits from these drugs in pregnancy may be acceptable despite potential risks.

Children

Lamotrigine has been used in children and young teenagers in other countries, but because of the higher risk of fatal side effects in children, lamotrigine is only approved for use in patients over age 18. Topiramate has been recently approved by the FDA for use in children.

Older Patients

Older patients seem to manage about the same as younger patients on lamotrigine, topiramate, and olanzapine, but there is little experience with using these medications in older patients with psychiatric problems.

Advantages

These drugs offer real hope to those people with bipolar disorders who have not been able to obtain relief from lithium and/or antidepressants. In addition, the weight loss often triggered by topiramate can be useful for patients who have gained a little weight while taking mood stabilizers. In some studies, between 20 and 50 percent of patients taking topiramate lost weight.

Disadvantages

Because these drugs have only been available for a short time, there is no information about long-term side effects; their use with mood disorders is even more recent. It isn't known if people who do well at first on these drugs will continue to flourish after many years of treatment. In addition, topiramate increases the likelihood of developing kidney stones (which may be prevented by drinking lots of water).

Conclusion

We've seen how lithium and Zyprexa can be of great help in the treatment of manic-depression, especially early in the course of the disease. However, some experts believe that manic-depression is a progressive disease that may worsen to the point where lithium just doesn't work anymore.

Even the alternative treatments (Tegretol and Depakote) may not fully control the symptoms of the disease in every person. For people like Jack, who was introduced at the beginning of this chapter, hope lies in the future, in some new drug that scientists may even now be testing. In the next chapter we'll discuss the herbal alternatives to antidepressants—St. John's wort and SAM-e.

8

HERBAL ANTIDEPRESSANTS

"I tried all the medicines my doctor recommended for depression. None worked and each had side effects, so I asked my doctor if we could try St. John's wort. He was more surprised than I was when it worked out so well."
— Nancy, 42

To ward off evil, Germans hung St. John's wort over their doorways. Pre-Christians stuffed it into amulets around their necks, and even St. Columba himself hid a branch of the herb inside his robes. It was whispered that the plant could make warlocks fly and fend off the evil eye. And for 2,000 years, St. John's wort (*Hypericum perforatum*) has been used by herbal healers for its antidepressant qualities.

Ancient physicians Hippocrates (460–377 B.C.), Dioscorides (A.D. 41–68), Galen (A.D. 150–200), and Pliny (A.D. 23–79) all used St. John's wort as a treatment for menstrual disorders. By the Middle Ages, herbalists were prescribing it for depression and anxiety, and in the mid-nineteenth century, the Shakers (master herbalists and giants of the mail-order seed business) sold St. John's wort as a cure for "low spirits."

St. John's wort includes any species of the large and widespread genus *Hypericum*, a sturdy perennial weed with yellow, five-petal flowers. In the rangelands of the American West, it's known as "noxious weed"—the bane of cowboys because it competed with native plants and threatened grazing livestock with potentially toxic side effects of fatal sun sensitivity.

The plant's size varies enormously, from the tiny, 4-inch matted *Hypericum anagalloides* (bog St. John's wort) to the towering *H. perforatum*, which can reach 32 feet tall. It's this giant form that is used to treat depression, not its attractive cousin most often sold in nurseries. Each of the lanced leaves of *H. perforatum* is covered with tiny purple-black dots containing hypericin, which is responsible for the reddish stain that results when you rub the foliage against your skin. It has a peculiar odor and a bitter, astringent taste.

St. John's wort is one of the most thoroughly researched medicinal herbs. Most of the studies have been done in Germany and other European countries, and all found the plant to be safe with few side effects. In fact, in more than 2,000 years of use, there has never been a recorded human death related to this plant—as opposed to aspirin, which kills about 500 people a year in overdose. Millions of Europeans use St. John's wort to treat chronic depression; one German brand is prescribed at a rate of seven to one over Prozac.

How St. John's Wort Works

When used daily for at least a month, St. John's wort seems to help mildly depressed people regain overall mental balance, normalizing mood and mental attitude. Exactly how it manages to do this is unclear, but European studies have found it is more effective than placebo and as effective as some older antidepressants.

In response to the public clamor over the plant, the United States launched the first clinical trial in 1997 comparing St. John's wort with SSRIs in the treatment of moderate depression. The three-year study, sponsored by the National Institute of Mental Health, the Office of Alternative Medicine, and the Office of Dietary Supplements, included 336 patients with major depression randomly assigned in an eight-week trial to one of three treatments (St. John's wort, an SSRI such as Prozac or Paxil, or placebo). Researchers hope that the study will provide solid answers about whether St. John's wort works as well as the best antidepressants for clinical depression. The study is the first rigorous clinical trial of the herb that is large enough and long enough to fully determine whether it works, according to NIMH director, Steven Hyman, M.D.

An overview of 23 clinical trials in Europe, published in an August 1996 issue of the *British Medical Journal,* found that the herb may be useful in cases of mild to moderate depression. Scientists who analyzed data from these randomized trials found that St. John's wort was much more effective than a placebo. Its response rates are similar to (or even slightly better than) older antidepressants—without the significant potential side effects. The plant was also better tolerated than traditional antidepressant drugs.

One of the most impressive studies was conducted in Austria, with 105 men and women diagnosed with depressive symptoms. Half the patients took a 300-milligram dose three times a day for a month; the other half took a sugar pill prepared to look and taste like the herbal extract. All the patients were tested for depression every two weeks. Two-thirds of those taking St. John's wort responded with a 50 percent decrease in depression. They reported that they were sleeping better and noted improvements in feelings of sadness, hopelessness, helplessness, and uselessness.

Although encouraging, this European research still left some unanswered questions about exactly how the herb works, explained Wayne Jonas, M.D., director of OAM. Despite the huge number of European studies, none looked at long-term use. Furthermore, published studies have used several different doses, which makes it hard to compare findings.

Scientists suspect that the reddish pigment, hypericin, contained in St. John's wort is primarily responsible for boosting mood through its action on the chemistry of the brain, affecting serotonin and dopamine by interfering with the breakdown of neurotransmitters. It is unclear whether whole plant extracts are more effective antidepressants than is hypericin alone.

Side Effects

One of the benefits of St. John's wort that herbalists cite is its apparent mild side effect profile. A few people feel nauseated when taking the drug on an empty stomach. Animal studies suggests that taking large amounts of the herb may make the skin more sensitive to the sun.

If you're sensitive to caffeine, St. John's wort may make you a bit nervous or anxious (especially if you combine caffeine with the herb). After all, many scientists believe St. John's wort is chemically similar to Prozac, and Prozac can trigger anxious feelings in certain patients.

Some studies suggest that St. John's wort may interfere with a key drug used in AIDS cocktails, as well as a drug used for transplant patients. Two studies published in *The Lancet* found that St. John's wort dulls the effectiveness of both the HIV medicine indinavir and the transplant drug cyclosporin. The FDA is working with drug manufacturers to insert a caution against using the herb with these drugs. Although both studies only used a few participants, the strength of the findings meant the results were significant.

Some scientists also believe the herb can have an effect on anesthesia during an operation. If you are about to undergo elective surgery, you should tell your anesthesiologist if you have taken St. John's wort within the past two weeks.

However, many of the side effects (especially the milder ones) disappear after the body adjusts to the herb. It may help to decrease the dosage until you become accustomed to St. John's wort.

Of course, if you do experience severe unpleasant side effects, you should consult your health care provider immediately and stop taking the herb. All symptoms should cease within a few days after the last dose is taken.

Drug Interactions

You should never take St. John's wort with any other antidepressant, especially an MAOI or an SSRI.

Because St. John's wort may be quite similar to an SSRI, you should always wait at least two weeks before stopping the herb and starting an MAOI (and vice versa).

Some anesthesiologists recommend that anyone contemplating surgery that requires anesthesia should stop taking the herb two weeks before the procedure. At least a few studies have suggested that St. John's wort may act in ways similar to an MAOI, and MAOIs can cause problems with anesthesia. Until research has definitively proven the exact chemical action of St. John's wort, it's better to be safe.

How Much Should You Take?

According to research, the most effective dosage is 300 milligrams of the hypericum extract three times a day, for a total of 900 milligrams. Most people do well when taking the herb in the morning, as soon as they get up, with the second dose about three hours later, and the final dose three hours after that. Others prefer taking two doses at breakfast and a third at lunch. Most experts recommend taking St. John's wort early in the day so as not to interfere with sleep—a problem some people have with the herb. Since the side effects are rare even in significantly higher doses, you can take four 250-milligram capsules a day, if the only herb you can find occurs in this amount.

Herbalists don't recommend more than 300 milligrams a day for children or the elderly, but no studies have been done on the safety of this herb for use in children.

After six weeks, you should evaluate how you're doing on the 900-milligrams-a-day schedule. (It may take this long to notice an effect, just as it can take weeks to notice the effects of antidepressant drugs.) Studies indicate that it can take hypericum longer to reach its full effectiveness than prescription antidepressants (antidepressants themselves may take as long as a month to begin working).

If you feel that you have not responded to St. John's wort, then you should consult your doctor and discuss taking a prescription antidepressant instead. Not everyone responds to St. John's wort, just as not everyone responds to antidepressants. It's very important not to decide after a week or two that the herb just isn't helping your depression.

Forms of St. John's Wort

This herb is available as a standardized tablet or capsule, oil, extract, spray, and essence. You can also buy dried leaves with which to make a tea, or grow the herb yourself.

> ➤ *Tablets:* This is the form most people take and the easiest to find. Tablets are available at most drugstores, discount department stores, and food stores. Some brands are made from standardized extracts. Look for 300-milligram tablets standardized to 0.3 percent. Take one tablet three times a day.

> ➤ *Oil:* Good quality oils are available at natural food stores. Look for bottles with a rich, red color liquid; that signifies the compound was made when the flowers were freshest. The oil will keep up to two years if stored in a dark place.

> ➤ *Extract:* An extract of St. John's wort is the best choice for treating mild depression and fighting

viruses. Commercial extracts are standardized to 0.05 percent hypericin. For correct dosage, follow the directions on the bottle.

➤ *Spray:* Oral spray versions of St. John's wort were approved in May 2000. The spray is aimed under the tongue or inside the cheek for instant absorption directly into the bloodstream, bypassing the stomach.

➤ *Tinctures:* Several brands are available in natural food stores. Read the label to make sure it was harvested in the wild. A safe dose is 40 drops of tincture, three times daily.

When buying St. John's wort (or any botanical), keep these tips in mind:

➤ Buy from only reliable sources.

➤ Make sure the product is standardized.

➤ Make sure the product is dated, and throw away anything expired.

➤ Avoid extra-large doses.

➤ Don't use St. John's wort for serious conditions without the advice or supervision of a qualified health practitioner.

➤ Don't use St. John's wort (or any herb) during pregnancy or while breast-feeding without the approval of your doctor.

➤ Don't use St. John's wort with any other anti-depressant, or combine with *any* other drug (including nonprescription drugs) without the advice of your doctor.

Also, be aware that St. John's wort is considered a supplement, not a drug. The FDA does not regulate the herb; therefore, it is not checked for either contents or potency. This means that a product may or may not contain what the label indicates. Manufacturers can legally call a product "hypericum" or "St. John's wort" even if it contains a tiny quantity of the herb.

St. John's Wort and the Elderly

People over age 65 and those who are chronically or severely ill are more likely than others to suffer from depression. Unfortunately, the same people are more susceptible to the side effects of traditional antidepressants. In other cases, conventional antidepressants may interact unpleasantly with other medications the elderly are already taking. For these reasons, St. John's wort may be particularly helpful, since the rare side effects are not serious in most cases.

SAM-e

SAM-e is another natural antidepressant. It is not an herb, hormone, vitamin, or any type of nutrient, but a stabilized, synthetic form of S-adenosylmethionine (SAM), a chemical produced naturally in all animals. In the human body, SAM-e is known to be essential to at least 35 biochemical processes, including maintaining the structure of cell membranes and manufacturing substances vital to transmitting nerve impulses and influencing emotions and moods. SAM-e reportedly works to ease depression by boosting dopamine and serotonin neurotransmitter metabolism and receptor function, and possibly repairing myelin which surrounds nerve cells. Some studies of SAM-e found it to be an effective treatment for mild to moderate depression, acting faster than tricyclic anti-depressants such as imipramine (Tofranil).

The substance was introduced to the United States from Italy and received plenty of publicity, including enthusiastic articles in *Newsweek,* media coverage, promo-tional books, full-page ads in newspapers, and numerous Web sites. Proponents believe SAM-e is an effective treat-ment for depression, arthritis, and liver disease. Like other supplements, it not regulated by the FDA.

The potential benefits and risks of SAM-e remain unclear. In Europe it is sold as a prescription drug for arthritis, depression, and liver disease, but in the United States it is available without prescription. One potential problem with SAM-e is that it is converted into homo-cysteine in the body, and high levels of homocysteine may raise the risk of heart disease. Critics are concerned that SAM-e may promote excessive levels of homocysteine. Marketers of SAM-e recommend a daily dose of 400 mil-ligrams, but there is no standardized dose in the current market. In addition, raw SAM-e is said to degrade quickly unless stored at proper temperatures; there is no guarantee that pills in the store have been properly handled. SAM-e is very expensive; a daily dose can cost anywhere from $2.50 to $18.

For healthy people SAM-e has no value, so it shouldn't be taken as a tonic or mood booster. It does not prevent any known disorder, and it will not repair the liver damage caused by heavy drinking. Side effects include stomach upset and other gastrointestinal problems.

Two brands of SAM-e (Nature Made and GNC) are imported from the original manufacturer in Italy in enteric-coated tablets which protect the compound from breaking down. In Italy, SAM-e is so popular it outsells Prozac.

Conclusion

In this chapter, you've learned about alternatives to traditional antidepressants that may be an option for people with mild symptoms of depression. In the next chapter, you'll read about some of the newest treatments currently being studied.

9
In the Future

"I'm lithium-resistant and I don't respond very well to Tegretol or Depakote, so my only hope is for some new drug to be developed to treat manic-depression. I don't care about side effects or what the drug might do 10 years from now. I need help now."

—Gerry, 53

The treatment of depression has come a long way in the past 40 years, but there are still problems to be overcome. Still needed are antidepressants with even fewer side effects and medications that will help the small percentage of depressed people who don't respond to any drug.

People like Gerry are counting on drug companies to come up with another "miracle drug"—like Prozac and the SSRIs—that will address his manic-depression. He has good reason to be hopeful.

Analysts predict that in the new millennium, the market for antidepressants will double to more than $6 billion. Pharmaceutical manufacturers are poised on the brink of a virtual flood of new antidepressants ready to join today's $3-billion antidepressant market. New medicines are currently being tested for mood disorders. But that doesn't mean they'll all be on the market in the near future.

How a Drug Is Born

On average, it takes 12 years for an experimental drug to travel from the laboratory to your medicine chest. Only 5 out of every 5,000 compounds that are initially tested make it to human testing; only one of these five is ever approved for human use.

The U.S. system of drug approvals is among the most stringent in the world, and it usually costs a company about $359 million to shepherd one medicine from the laboratory to the pharmacy. The first step in the journey from drug lab to pharmacy shelf is preclinical testing, in which a drug company conducts animal and lab safety studies and determines how the compound works against a particular disease. These tests take about three-and-a-half years.

After completing this phase, a company files an "investigational new drug application" with the FDA for permission to test the drug on humans. The application shows the results of the preclinical testing and describes details about the upcoming studies, how the compound works, and any possible toxic effects. Once the application is approved, progress reports on clinical trials must be submitted yearly.

Next comes the year-long Phase I of the clinical trials in which 20 to 80 healthy volunteers test the drug for safety and provide evidence of how the drug is absorbed, distributed, and excreted. Then comes about two years of Phase II effectiveness research involving between 100 and 300 volunteer patients who have the targeted disease. Phase III involves another three years of further tests of usefulness and side effects, and usually involves between 1,000 and 3,000 patients in clinics and hospitals.

Once all three phases of the clinical trials are over and the drug is considered to be safe and effective, the company files a New Drug Application (NDA), a document of more than 100,000 pages packed with all the scientific data the company has gathered. Although by law the FDA must review the NDA within six months, the average review for approved compounds takes about 26.5 months.

Once the FDA approves a new drug's application, the new medicine becomes available for doctors to prescribe. However, the drug company's job isn't over. It must still submit periodic reports to the FDA, including any information about side effects as they become known. For some drugs, the FDA requires more studies (called Phase IV) to evaluate long-term effects.

Once a drug is approved to treat a disease, physicians don't always prescribe it only for its approved use. For example, Prozac was initially approved just for the treatment of depression, but today physicians prescribe it for disorders ranging from migraines to shyness.

Upcoming Antidepressants

Ten years ago, scientists suspected that there were two or three different ways to influence serotonin function. Today, researchers believe there may be at least 14 different serotonin receptors, and they are currently developing

HOW TO JOIN A CLINICAL
ANTIDEPRESSANT TRIAL

If you've not found relief with any antidepressant, including tricyclics, MAOIs, and SSRIs, you have one final recourse: participating in a new anti-depressant trial. Participation is free, and you'll receive close attention from highly qualified doctors during the trial.

➤ First step: Locate upcoming drug trial in radio, TV, or print ads.

➤ Telephone investigator for brief phone screening interview.

➤ If you're acceptable, you'll participate in a detailed psychiatric interview followed by a medical exam (including EKG).

➤ If eligible, you'll be asked to sign a two-page informed consent document.

➤ Phase I studies: Inpatients are treated with drugs in their earliest stage of development to determine dosages and safety.

➤ Phase II studies: Both in- and outpatients are given differing doses to check efficacy, tolerance, and side effects.

➤ Phase III studies: The new drug is compared to a placebo and one or two standard drugs.

➤ Phase IV: Drug studies take place after marketing to investigate the drug's usefulness with other diseases.

compounds that either block or stimulate these receptors in different patterns. Using DNA technology, scientists can isolate one receptor and screen it to see which chemical affects it. This way, the industry can identify potential drugs that specifically act on one serotonin receptor and avoid receptors associated with unpleasant side effects.

For example, scientists are searching for an SSRI that doesn't affect the 5HT3 receptor, which would eliminate the side effect of nausea.

Other scientists are trying to combine medications in new ways for even greater treatment benefits, such as combining Paxil, Zoloft, or Prozac with the beta-blocker pindolol (Visken) in an attempt to block the serotonin 1A receptors, which might boost the antidepressant effects of SSRIs.

Edronax (Reboxetine) and Other Noradrenaline Reuptake Inhibitors (NARIs). These antidepressants selectively block the return of the neurotransmitter noradrenaline (norepinephrine) to carry messages to various parts of the brain. A lack of norepinephrine is linked to the decreased energy, interest, and motivation found in depressed patients. Studies have shown that the NARIs are at least as effective as the tricyclic antidepressants and SSRIs in treating major depressive disorders. However, some studies suggest that Edronax and other NARIs aren't as effective as SSRIs in the treatment of obsessive-compulsive disorder or panic disorder.

The side effect profile of the NARIs is preferable to the tricyclics. NARIs cause less nausea and sexual dysfunction than the SSRIs. The most common side effects of the NARIs are dry mouth, insomnia, constipation, increased sweating, and rapid heartbeat. These symptoms tend to improve over time. Also some preliminary work indicates that combining NARIs with SSRIs or MAOIs may be extremely useful in treatment-resistant depression.

Neurokinin-1 Receptors. Another totally new class of antidepressants may block the neurokinin-1 (NK-1) receptor; these drugs, which were first studied for pain and anxiety control, are now being researched as an antidepressant.

Dopamine. Scientists are looking at dopamine as a possible link to depression, since this neurotransmitter is affected by some of the MAOIs currently on the market. Scientists suspect that dopamine may be particularly associated with atypical depression and bipolar disorder.

Flesinoxan. Flesinoxan (Solvay Pharmaceuticals) affects the serotonin receptors and is currently in Phase III trials, where it appears to be effective and well-tolerated. Most common side effects reported with Flesinoxan were nausea (11 percent) and dizziness (7 percent).

Sunepitron. This drug selectively blocks the serotonin (5-HT) receptor as well as the alpha-2 receptor. Early clinical trials have found that it works both for generalized anxiety and major depression. Side effects include headache, nausea, and insomnia. Pfizer is currently conducting Phase III clinical trials.

Survector (Amineptine). This new—and yet unapproved—tricyclic is a relatively selective dopamine reuptake blocker that at higher doses also boosts the release of dopamine. This mild psychostimulant is a fast-acting mood brightener that may sometimes cause spontaneous orgasms. Unlike other tricyclics, it doesn't interfere with sex drive or thinking abilities. It is considered to have abuse potential.

Aurorex (Moclobemide). This reversible inhibitor of monoamine oxidase type A (RIMAs) is among a new group of antidepressants that are more selective and reversible than older MAOIs. As a result, the severe dietary restrictions that must be observed when taking MAOIs aren't necessary with RIMAs. Aurorex is as effective as tricyclics with fewer side effects and is currently widely available outside the United States. Studies suggest that the drug is significantly more effective than placebo and at least comparable to the SSRIs. Higher doses may improve effectiveness for more severe depression.

INN 00835. INN 00835 is a member of a new class of peptide antidepressants that appears to have a rapid onset of action within three to five days, peaking between one and two weeks. There appears to be little drug-related adverse effects with INN 00835, which is currently in Phase II and III clinical trials.

Substance P Blockers. Merck is currently pursuing several substance P blockers, which appear to work fairly well. A number of other companies, including Pfizer and Eli Lilly, are also working on substance P blockers.

Conclusion

The only thing more tragic than the thousands of depressed people is the fact that so many aren't being treated for their disorder. Far too many Americans still fear the stigma of the label of mental illness. Some still believe that all antidepressants will make them dopey or groggy. And many refuse to seek a psychiatrist's help, feeling that being "a little down" is a moral weakness and not a physiological disorder.

With the new antidepressants that have already been discovered, and the new preparations currently under investigation, there is no reason for any depressed person not to have a chance at a normal, healthy life.

GLOSSARY

adrenergic   Referring to the activation of neurons by catecholamine transmitters (such as epinephrine, norepinephrine, and dopamine).

agitated depression   A major depressive disorder characterized by restlessness, insomnia, and loss of appetite.

alprazolam   The generic name for Xanax, a benzodiazepine tranquilizer that may be useful for short-term treatment of minor depression.

amantadine   The generic name of Symmetrel.

amine   Organic compounds containing the amino group ($-NH_2$).

amino acids   Any organic acid containing one or more amino ($-NH_2$) groups; a basic part of proteins and the basic building blocks of neurotransmitters.

Anafranil   The brand name for clomipramine, a tricyclic antidepressant (also prescribed for obsessive-compulsive disorder).

anhedonia   Inability to experience pleasure from activities that usually produce pleasurable feelings.

antagonist   A drug that reduces or blocks the action of another drug.

anticholinergic effects The interference with the action of acetylcholine in the brain and peripheral nervous system by any drug. This term is often used to refer to the side effects of tricyclic antidepressants, such as dry mouth, blurred vision, and constipation.

antidepressant A medication used to treat depression.

anxiety A feeling of apprehension, worry, or distress (often about events in the future); there may also be breathing problems, racing heartbeat, trembling, and sweating.

Artane The brand name of trihexyphenidyl, a muscle relaxant used to treat Parkinsonism.

Asendin The brand name of amoxapine, a tricyclic antidepressant.

Ativan The brand name of lorazepam, an antianxiety medication also prescribed for anxiety with depression.

atypical bipolar II depression A clinical condition in which periods of major depression alternate with periods of mild elation.

atypical depression A type of depression in which the person reacts to the environment, is sensitive to rejection, and may gain weight and sleep more than usual; this condition is the opposite of typical depression, which is characterized by weight loss and insomnia.

Aventyl The brand name of nortriptyline, a tricyclic antidepressant.

barbiturate A habit-forming drug used to induce sleep or treat anxiety.

behavior therapy   A form of psychotherapy that seeks to modify behavior by manipulating the environment and behavior.

Benadryl   A nonprescription antihistamine used to treat allergies; it is also used to treat Parkinsonism.

benzodiazepines   A class of psychotropic drugs that have a hypnotic and sedative action, used mainly as tranquilizers for the control of symptoms due to anxiety or stress and as a sleeping aid for insomnia.

binge eating disorder   Episodic uncontrolled eating of large amounts of food without the purging that characterizes bulimia (binge-purge eating disorder).

biogenic amine hypothesis   The concept that abnormalities in the biogenic amines (especially the neurotransmitters norepinephrine, dopamine, and serotonin) are involved in depression. The idea was developed when researchers noticed that monoamine oxidase inhibitors and some tricyclic drugs were able to improve mood by affecting certain brain monoamine functions.

biogenic amines   Organic substances subdivided into catecholamines (epinephrine, dopamine, and norepinephrine) and indoles (tryptophan and serotonin), all of which appear to play a role in the development of depression.

bipolar disorder   A major affective disorder characterized by both mania and depression. A mild form of this disorder is sometimes called "cyclothymia." Bipolar disorders may be divided into manic, depressed, or mixed types on the basis of the patient's symptoms.

Manic type   Symptoms are characterized by excitement, euphoria, expansive or irritable mood, hyperactivity, pressured speech, flight of ideas, limited sleep needs, distractibility, impaired judgment. There may be grandiose or elated delusions.

Depressed type   Symptoms are characterized by slow thinking, lowered mood, decreased movement or agitation, loss of interest, guilt, negative self-esteem, sleep problems, and appetite loss.

Mixed type   Symptoms of mania and depression occur at the same time.

bipolar I disorder   Also known as manic-depression, this is a clinical condition characterized by alternating episodes of major depression and mania or elation often severe enough to require hospitalization.

bipolar II disorder   A clinical condition characterized by alternating periods of major depression and mild mania. A patient may need to be hospitalized during depressed periods but usually not during the manic phase.

bipolar III disorder   A term used to describe a depressed person who develops mild or severe mania only after taking certain drugs (such as antidepressants).

bupropion   The generic name for Wellbutrin, an antidepressant drug.

BuSpar   The brand name of buspirone, a nonhabit-forming antianxiety medication.

buspirone   The generic name for BuSpar, a nonhabit-forming antianxiety medication.

carbamazepine   The generic name for Tegretol.

Celexa   The brand name for citalopram HBr, an SSRI antidepressant.

chloral hydrate   The generic name for Noctec, a sleeping medication.

chlorpromazine   The generic name for Thorazine.

cholinergic   Activated by acetylcholine.

citalopram   The generic name for the SSRI Celexa.

clinical depression   A medical term often used for major depression.

clomipramine   The generic name for Anafranil, a tricyclic antidepressant.

clonidine   An antihypertensive (high blood pressure) drug also used for narcotic withdrawal.

Cogentin   The brand name for benztropine, a medication used to treat Parkinsonism.

cognitive therapy   A structured form of short-term psychotherapy in which the goal is to change negative, inaccurate ways of thinking.

Coumadin   The brand name for warfarin, a blood-thinning medication.

cyclothymia   A form of manic-depression characterized by relatively mild highs and lows.

Cytomel   A thyroid hormone sometimes used to boost the effectiveness of an antidepressant.

Dalmane The brand name of flurazepam, a benzodiazepine drug used as a hypnotic agent or sleeping pill.

Depakote The brand name for valproic acid, an anticonvulsant drug and an alternative to lithium for the treatment of manic-depression.

Deprenyl A European monoamine oxidase inhibitor that lacks the "cheese effect" (harmful interaction with cheese and other tyramine-containing foods), which is used to treat Parkinson's disease.

depressive illness Depression characterized by depressed mood (sadness, hopelessness, etc.), reduced energy level (fatigue, loss of interest, etc.), and negative self-image. Common features include sleep problems, early awakening, loss of appetite, etc.

depressive reaction A reactive depression that represents an understandable response to a significant loss or stressful life situation, involving a sense of despondency and distress. It is usually comparatively mild to moderate and usually passes within two weeks to six months.

desipramine The generic name for Norpramin, a tricyclic antidepressant.

Desyrel The brand name for trazodone, an antidepressant structurally unlike the tricyclics, MAOIs, and SSRIs.

diazepam The generic name for Valium.

dopamine One of the major neurotransmitters found in the synapses of the brain; low levels of dopamine are associated with depression.

double depression An episode of major depression that occurs in addition to a chronic, long-term mild depression.

DSM-IV An abbreviation for the fourth edition of the *Diagnostic and Statistical Manual of Mental Disorders* published by the American Psychiatric Association. *DSM-IV* lists all symptoms for all psychiatric disorders.

dysphoria An unpleasant mood associated with a shifting set of symptoms including sadness, anxiety, and irritability.

dysthymic disorder This mild but persistent form of depression is also called "depressive neurosis," a chronic disturbance of mood involving depression *for at least two years* (one year in children). In addition, symptoms include poor appetite or overeating, insomnia or excessive fatigue, low energy, poor self-esteem, poor concentration, and hopelessness.

Effexor The brand name for venlafaxine, an anti-depressant.

elation A strong feeling of exhilaration, euphoria, and optimism.

Elavil The brand name for amitriptyline, a tricyclic antidepressant.

endogenous depression A spontaneous, unexplained, and seemingly unprovoked depression of moderate to severe degree.

epinephrine Also known as adrenaline, this is one of the catecholamines secreted by the adrenal gland and the sympathetic nervous system responsible for physical symptoms of fear and anxiety.

fluoxetine The generic name for Prozac, an SSRI antidepressant.

fluvoxamine The generic name for Luvox, an SSRI antidepressant.

generic drugs A drug not controlled by a manufacturer's trademark.

Halcion The brand name for triazolam, a short-acting benzodiazepine hypnotic or sleeping pill.

Haldol The brand name for haloperidol, an antipsychotic drug.

hyperthymia A mood characterized by high energy, confidence, and activity; it is more energetic than a normal mood but less than mild forms of mania (hypomania).

hypomania A mildly elevated mood lasting a few days, less intense than mania but more intense than hyperthymia.

hypothalamus A part of the brain responsible for regulating automatic activities of the body, such as hunger, thirst, body temperature, and sexual desire.

imipramine The generic name for Tofranil, a tricyclic antidepressant.

interpersonal psychotherapy A type of structured short-term therapy designed to treat depression.

Lamictal The brand name for lamotrigine, a mood-stabilizing anticonvulsant used to treat resistant bipolar disorder (manic-depression).

lamotrigine   The generic name for Lamictal, a mood-stabilizing anticonvulsant used to treat resistant bipolar disorder (manic-depression).

levodopa   The precursor of dopamine; as a drug, this is used to treat Parkinson's disease.

Librium   The brand name for chlordiazepoxide, an antianxiety drug and member of the benzodiazepine family.

lithium   An element which, when used as a medication, can stabilize fluctuating ups and downs of mood disorders by shifting the levels of water and electrolytes.

L-tryptophan   An amino acid used to make serotonin.

Ludiomil   The brand name for maprotiline, a tetracyclic antidepressant.

Luvox   The brand name for fluvoxamine, an SSRI antidepressant.

major affective disorder   A group of disorders with a persistent, prominent disturbance of mood (depression or mania) and a full syndrome of symptoms; major depression and bipolar disorder are both examples of major affective disorder.

major depressive episode   Also known as clinical or unipolar depression, or major depressive disorder, this is an episode lasting at least two weeks, characterized by at least four of the following symptoms: loss of ability to experience pleasure and interest, fatigue, feelings of worthlessness or guilt, concentration problems, appetite and sleep disturbances, frequent thoughts of suicide and death. If at least four of these symptoms are present *in addition* to at least one episode of mania, then the diagnosis becomes bipolar disorder (or manic-depressive illness).

mania A period of persistent elation characterized by hyperactivity, agitation, rapid talking, excitement, or flight of ideas.

manic-depressive illness A disorder characterized by alternating episodes of moderate to severe depression and unstable periods of elation. It is also known as bipolar I disorder. The periods of mania are distinct, with a predominant mood that is elevated, expansive, or irritable. Other symptoms of mania include hyperactivity, flight of ideas, inflated self-esteem, little need for sleep, distractibility, and excessive involvement in activities that may be flamboyant, bizarre, or disorganized.

MAOI Monoamine oxidase inhibitor.

maprotiline The generic name for Ludiomil, a tetracyclic antidepressant.

masked depression A type of depression hidden behind physical symptoms with no apparent physical cause.

melancholia A term used to refer to a severe form of depression. In psychiatric diagnoses, "major depression with melancholia" refers to a severe depression including loss of pleasure, worse morning moods, psychomotor retardation or agitation, weight loss, and insomnia.

Mellaril The brand name for thioridazine, an antipsychotic drug used rarely for the short-term treatment of depression with anxiety.

metabolite The chemical compound produced by the breakdown of a drug in the body.

methylphenidate (Ritalin) Drug often used to treat hyperactive children that may be tried for long-term treatment of selected elderly people with depression.

MHPG (3-methoxy-4-hydroxyphenylglycol) A major metabolite of norepinephrine excreted in urine; low MHPG levels occur in depression, while high levels are found in bipolar patients during manic phases. Research suggests that MHPG levels may be used to classify depression types and to predict responses to tricyclic antidepressants.

Mianserin A tetracyclic antidepressant available in Europe but not yet approved for use in the United States.

mirtazapine The generic name for the antidepressant Remeron.

monoamine oxidase (MAO) An enzyme that breaks down biogenic amines (neurotransmitters). Inhibition of this enzyme by certain antidepressant drugs (MAO inhibitors) may relieve a patient's depression.

monoamine oxidase inhibitor (MAOI) A class of antidepressants that keeps the enzyme monoamine oxidase from breaking down, resulting in higher levels of norepinephrine and serotonin at the nerve synapses.

mood (affective) disorders   A group of clinical conditions characterized by feelings of lack of control over mood or emotions, primarily depression, and mania. Mood disorders can affect basic functions such as cognitive ability, sleep patterns, appetite, and sexuality, and can interfere with personal and professional life.

mood episode   A mood syndrome that has no known organic cause and that is not part of a psychotic disorder (such as schizophrenia). A mood episode can be either major depressive, manic, or hypomanic.

mood syndrome   A group of mood and associated symptoms that occur together for a minimum amount of time. Mood syndromes can occur as part of a mood disorder, a psychotic disorder, or an organic mental disorder.

Nardil   The brand name for phenelzine, an MAOI antidepressant.

nefazadone   The generic name for the antidepressant Serzone.

neuron   A nerve cell.

neurotransmitter   A chemical in the nervous system (such as dopamine or serotonin) that carries messages across the gaps (synapses) between neurons. Dysfunction in this neurotransmitter system has been linked to depression.

norepinephrine   Also called noradrenaline, this is one of the three major neurotransmitters found in the brain and implicated in the development of depression. High levels of this substance in the brain have been linked to manic states; low levels have been linked to depression.

norfluoxetine   A metabolite of Prozac.

normal reactive depression   A short-term depression caused by grief or bereavement.

Norpramin   The brand name for desipramine, a tricyclic antidepressant.

nortriptyline   The generic name for the tricyclic antidepressants Pamelor and Aventyl.

obsessive-compulsive disorder   A clinical condition characterized by distressing repetition of thoughts that are intense, frightening, absurd, or unusual, together with ritualized actions that are usually bizarre and irrational.

olanzapine   The generic name for Zyprexa, a schizophrenia drug used for the short-term treatment of acute mania.

orthostatic hypotension   A precipitous fall in blood pressure upon sitting or standing up, causing dizziness or fainting. This is a common side effect in some antidepressants.

Pamelor   The brand name for nortriptyline, a tricyclic antidepressant.

Parnate   The brand name for tranylcypromine, an MAOI antidepressant.

paroxetine   The generic name for Paxil, an SSRI antidepressant.

Paxil   The brand name for paroxetine, an SSRI antidepressant.

phenelzine   The generic name for Nardil, an MAOI antidepressant.

phenothiazine   A generic name for a family of antipsychotic drugs including Thorazine, Stelazine, and Mellaril.

protriptyline   The generic name for Vivactil, a tricyclic antidepressant.

Prozac   The trade name for fluoxetine, an SSRI antidepressant.

psychotropic drugs   Medications that affect mood or mental activity.

rapid cyclers   Manic-depressive people who experience more than four mood swings a year.

reboxetine   The generic name for Vestra, one of a class of antidepressants known as the selective norepinephrine reuptake inhibitors (SNRIs). Also, the generic name for Edronax, a noradrenaline reuptake inhibitor (NARI).

Remeron   The brand name for mirtazapine, a new antidepressant that works on norepinephrine and serotonin.

SAM-e   An antidepressant supplement made from a synthetic form of S-adenosylmethionine, a natural chemical found in all animals.

selective norepinephrine reuptake inhibitor (SNRI) A class of antidepressants available in Europe since 1998 and granted an approval letter by the FDA in 1999. The class targets noradrenaline, which is deficient in some people with depression.

selective serotonin reuptake inhibitor (SSRI)   A class of antidepressants that work by blocking the reabsorption of serotonin in the brain, thus raising the levels of serotonin. SSRIs include Prozac, Celexa, Luvox, Zoloft, and Paxil.

serotonin   One of the three major neurotransmitters found in the synapses of the brain linked to the development of depression.

sertraline   The generic name for Zoloft, an SSRI antidepressant.

Serzone   The brand name for nefazadone, a serotonin-related antidepressant that is similar to an SSRI.

soft bipolar   A form of mania or hypomania that is too mild to meet the requirements of a formal *DSM-IV* diagnosis.

SNRI   Selective norepinephrine reuptake inhibitor.

SSRI   Selective serotonin reuptake inhibitor.

Stelazine   The brand name for trifluoperazine, a major antipsychotic or tranquilizer of the phenothiazine family.

subclinical depression   A form of depression not severe enough to meet the diagnostic criteria for major depression or dysthymia.

Surmontil   The brand name for trimipramine, a tricyclic antidepressant.

Survector   The brand name for amineptine, an antidepressant available in Europe.

synapse The gap between two nerve cells at which the transmission of nerve impulses occurs.

Tegretol The brand name for carbamazepine, an anticonvulsant drug and an alternative to lithium for the treatment of manic-depression.

tetracyclic antidepressant A class of antidepressants named for their four-ring chemical structure. Ludiomil is an example of a tetracyclic.

Tofranil The brand name for imipramine, the first tricyclic antidepressant.

Topamax The brand name for topiramate, a mood-stabilizing anticonvulsant drug used to treat bipolar disorder (manic-depression).

topiramate The generic name for Topamax, a mood-stabilizing anticonvulsant drug used to treat bipolar disorder (manic-depression).

tranylcypromine The generic name for Parnate, an MAOI antidepressant.

trazodone The generic name for Desyrel, an antidepressant.

treatment-resistant depression Depression that is not affected by any of the major classes of antidepressants.

tricyclic antidepressant A class of antidepressants named for their three-ring chemical structure. TCAs increase the level of norepinephrine and serotonin in the synapses of the brain.

unipolar psychoses Recurrent major depressions.

Valium The brand name of diazepam, an antianxiety medication and minor tranquilizer.

valproic acid The generic name for Depakote, an anticonvulsive medication used to treat manic-depression.

venlafaxine The generic name for Effexor, a new SNRI antidepressant.

vesicle A small saclike structure that forms the brain during fetal development.

Vestra The brand name for reboxetine, one of a class of antidepressants known as the selective norepinephrine reuptake inhibitors (SNRIs).

Vivactil The brand name for protriptyline, a tricyclic antidepressant.

Wellbutrin The brand name for bupropion, an antidepressant with a structure unlike SSRIs, MAOIs, or tricyclics.

withdrawal The process of stopping a drug.

Xanax The brand name for alprazolam, an antianxiety medication and minor tranquilizer.

Zoloft The brand name for sertraline, an SSRI antidepressant.

Zyprexa The brand name for olanzapine, a schizophrenia drug used for the short-term treatment of acute manic episodes associated with bipolar disorder (manic-depression).

REFERENCES

"ABCs of Antidepressants," *USA Today* 121 (February 1993): 12.

Ablow, Russell Keith. "Prozac: What Kind of Cure?" *Washington Post* 115 (February 11, 1992): WH9.

Ahmad, S. R. "USA: Fluoxetine 'Not Linked to Suicide,'" *The Lancet* 338 (October 5, 1951): 875–6.

Allhoff, T., et al. "Atrial Arrhythmia in a Woman Treated with Fluoxetine: Is There a Causal Relationship?" *Annals of Emergency Medicine* 37 (1): 116–7 (January 2001).

Askisal, H. S. "The Prevalent Clinical Spectrum of Bipolar Disorders: Beyond DSM-IV," *Journal of Clinical Psychopharmacology* 16 (April 1996): 4S–14S.

———, et al. "Fluoxetine Found Effective for Dysthymia," *Clinical Psychiatry News* 20 (2): 4F (February 1992).

———. "The Clinical Spectrum of So-Called 'Minor' Depressions," *American Journal of Psychotherapy* 46 (1): 9–22 (1992).

American Psychiatric Association. *Diagnostic and Statistical Manual of Mental Disorders IV-R*. Washington, D.C., 1994.

American Psychological Association. *Factsheet: Women and Depression*. Washington, D.C.

Angier, Natalie. "Can a Pill Called Prozac End Depression?" *Mademoiselle,* April 1990, 229–32.

Balon, Richard, et al. "Sexual Dysfunction During Antidepressant Treatment," *Journal of Clinical Psychiatry* 54 (June 1993): 67.

Barefoot, J. C., et al. "Depression and Long-Term Mortality Risk in Patients with Coronary Artery Disease," *American Journal of Cardiology* 78 (September 15, 1996): 613–17.

Baxter, Lewis R., et al. "Caudate Glucose Metabolic Rate Changes with Both Drug and Behavior Therapy for Obsessive-Compulsive Disorder," *Archives of General Psychiatry* 49 (1992): 681–89.

Beasley, C. M., et al. "Fluoxetine and Suicide: A Meta-analysis of Controlled Trials of Treatment for Depression," *British Medical Journal* 303 (1991): 685–92.

Begley, Sharon. "One Pill Makes You Larger, and One Pill Makes You Small," *Newsweek*, February 7, 1994, 36–40.

Berrettinni, Wade, et al. "X-Chromosome Markers and Manic-Depressive Illness," *Archives of General Psychiatry* 47 (April 1990): 366–73.

Bihm, B., and B. A. Wilson. "Understanding Fluoxetine (Prozac)," *Medsurgical Nursing* 5 (February 1996): 50–52, 56.

Bittman, B. J., and R. C. Young. "Mania in Elderly Men Treated with Bupropion," Letter, *American Journal of Psychiatry* 148 (4): 541 (1991).

Blondal, T., et al. "The Effects of Fluoxetine Combined with Nicotine Inhalers in Smoking Cessation—A Randomized Trial," *Addiction* 94 (7):1007–15 (July 1999).

Bloomfield, Harold, and Peter McWilliams. *How to Heal with Depression*, Los Angeles: Prelude Press, 1994.

Bohn, J., and J. W. Jefferson. *Lithium and Manic Depression: A Guide*, rev. ed. Madison, Wis.: Lithium Information Center, 1990.

Boulos, C., et al. "An Open Naturalistic Trial of Fluoxetine in Adolescents and Young Adults with Treatment-Resistant Major Depression," *Journal of Child and Adolescent Psychopharmacology* 2 (2): 103–111 (1992).

Bowe, Claudia. "Women and Depression: Are We Being Overdosed?" *Redbook*, March 1992, 42–5.

Bower, Bruce. "Drugs, Depression and Molecular Ferries," *Science News* 140 (October 26, 1991): 261.

Brandes, L. J., et al. "Stimulation of Malignant Growth in Rodents by Antidepressant Drugs at Clinically Relevant Doses," *Cancer Research* 52 (1992): 3796–3800.

Brendler, John, Michael Silver, Madlynn Haber, and John Sargent. *Madness, Chaos and Violence: Therapy with Families at the Brink.* New York: Basic Books, 1991.

Brodaty, Henry, et al. "Age and Depression," *Journal of Affective Disorders* 23 (1991): 137–49.

Brown, C., et al, "Treatment Outcomes for Primary Care Patients with Major Depression and Lifetime Anxiety Disorders," *American Journal of Psychiatry* 153 (October 1996): 1293–1300.

Burke, W. J., et al. "Weekly Dosing of Fluoxetine for the Continuation Phase of Treatment of Major Depression: Results of a Placebo-Controlled, Randomized Clinical Trial," *Journal of Clinical Psychopharmacology* 20 (4): 423–7 (August 2000).

Burns, David. *Feeling Good: The New Mood Therapy.* New York: Signet, 1980.

Cabrera-Vera, T. M., et al. "Effect of Prenatal Fluoxetine (Prozac) Exposure on Brain Serotonin Neurons in Prepubescent and Adult Male Rat Offspring," *Journal of Pharmacology Experimental Therapy* 280 (January 1997): 138–45.

Chilvers, C., et. al. "Antidepressant Drugs and Generic Counselling for Treatment of Major Depression in Primary Care: Randomised Trial with Patient Preference Arms," *British Medical Journal* 322 (7289): 772 (March 31, 2001).

Claxton, A., et al. "Patient Compliance to a New Enteric-Coated Weekly Formulation of Fluoxetine During Continuation Treatment of Major Depressive Disorder," *Journal of Clinical Psychiatry* 61 (12): 928–32 (December 2000).

Cohen, Bennet J., et al. "More Cases of SIADH with Fluoxetine," *American Journal of Psychiatry* 147 (7): 948–9 (July 1990).

Cohen, L. S., et al. "Birth Outcomes Following Prenatal Exposure to Fluoxetine," *Biological Psychiatry* 48 (10): 996–1000 (November 15, 2000).

"Committee Advises FDA on Antidepressants," *FDA Consumer* 25 (December 1991): 5.

Costa e Silva, et al. "Placebo-Controlled Study of Tianeptine in Major Depressive Episodes," *Neuropsychobiology* 35 (1997): 24–9.

Cowen, R. "Sociopaths, Suicide and Serotonin," *Science News* 136 (October 14, 1989): 250.

Cowley, Geoffrey. "The Culture of Prozac: How a Treatment for Depression Became as Familiar as Kleenex and as Socially Acceptable as Spring Water," *Newsweek*, February 7, 1994, 41–2.

———. "A Prozac Backlash: Does America's Favorite Antidepressant Make Some People Crazy?" *Newsweek*, April 1, 1991, 64–7.

———. "The Promise of Prozac," *Newsweek*, March 26, 1990, 38–41.

Cunningham, Malcolm, et al. "Eye Tics and Subjective Hearing Impairment During Fluoxetine Therapy," *American Journal of Psychiatry* 147 (7): 947–8 (July 1990).

Danish University Antidepressant Group. "Paroxetine: A Selective Serotonin Reuptake Inhibitor Showing Better Tolerance, but Weaker Antidepressant Effect Than Clomipramine in a Controlled Multicenter Study," *Journal of Affective Disorders* 18 (1990): 289–99.

Davis, Lori, et al. "Valproate as an Antidepressant in Major Depressive Disorder," *Psychopharmacology Bulletin* 32 (4): 647–52 (1996).

de Boer, T.H., et al. "Differences in Modulation of Noradrenergic and Serotonergic Transmission by the Alpha-2 Adrenoreceptor Antagonists, Mirtazapine, Mianserin and Idazoxan," *Journal of Pharmacological Experimental Therapy* 277 (May 1996): 852–60.

Delgado, Pedro, et al. "Serotonin Function and the Mechanism of Antidepressant Action: Reversal of Antidepressant-Induced Remission by Rapid Depletion of Plasma Tryptophan," *Archives of General Psychiatry* 47 (1990): 411–18.

Denniston, Philip, ed. *1993 Physicians' GenRX: Official Drug Reference of the FDA.* New York: Data Pharmaceutica, 1993.

"Depressing Danger," *Time,* May 17, 1993, 5.

Devlin, M. J., et al. "Open Treatment of Overweight Binge-Eaters with Phentermine and Fluoxetine as an Adjunct to Cognitive-Behavioral Therapy," *International Journal of Eating Disorders* 28 (3): 325–32 (November 2000).

Dittmann, R. W., et al. "Efficacy and Safety Findings from Naturalistic Fluoxetine Drug Treatment in Adolescent and Young Adult Patients," *Journal of Child and Adolescent Psychopharmacology* 10 (2): 91–102 (summer 2000).

Dowling, Colette. *You Mean I Don't Have to Feel This Way?* New York: Charles Scribner's Sons, 1991.

Duke, Patty. *A Brilliant Madness: Living with Manic-Depressive Illness.* New York: Bantam Books, 1992.

Eichelman, Burr. "Aggressive Behavior: From Laboratory to Clinic: Quo Vadit?" *Archives of General Psychiatry* 49 (6): 488–92 (June 1992).

Eisenberg, Leon. "Treating Depression and Anxiety in Primary Care: Closing the Gap Between Knowledge and Practice," *New England Journal of Medicine* 326 (1992): 1080–84.

Elmer-Dewitt, Philip. "Depression: The Growing Role of Drug Therapies," *Time,* July 6, 1992, 56–9.

Emptage, R. E., and T. P. Semia. "Depression in the Medically Ill Elderly; a Focus on Methylphenidate," *Annals of Pharmacotherapy* 30 (February 1996): 151–7.

Ekselitus, L., and L. von Knorring. "Effect on Sexual Function of Long-Term Treatment with Selective Serotonin Reuptake Inhibitors in Depressed Patients Treated in Primary Care," *Journal of Clinical Psychopharmacology* 21 (2): 154–60 (April 2001).

Falk, William. "Suit: Drug Prompted Suicide Attempts," *Newsday,* July 18, 1990, 8.

Fava, Maurizio, et al. "Fluoxetine versus Sertraline and Paroxetine in Major Depressive Disorder: Changes in Weight with Long-Term Treatment," *Journal of Clinical Psychiatry* 61 (11): 863–7 (November 2000).

———, et al. "Antidepressants Found to Prevent Depression-Related 'Anger Attacks,'" *Clinical Psychiatry News* (September 1992): 6.

———, and Jerold Rosenbaum. "Suicidality and Fluoxetine: Is There a Relationship?" *Journal of Clinical Psychiatry* 52 (March 1991): 108–111.

———. "Does Fluoxetine Increase the Risk of Suicide?" *The Harvard Mental Health Letter* 7 (7): 8 (January 1991).

Feder, R. "Fluoxetine-Induced Mania," *Journal of Clinical Psychiatry* 51 (12): 524–5 (1990).

Feighner, J. P. "A Comparative Trial of Fluoxetine and Amitriptyline in Patients with Major Depressive Disorder," *Journal of Clinical Psychiatry* 46 (1985): 369–72.

Ferguson, J. M. "The Effects of Antidepressants on Sexual Functioning in Depressed Patients: A Review," *Journal of Clinical Psychiatry* 62 (3) (suppl): 22–34 (2001).

———, et al. "Reemergence of Sexual Dysfunction in Patients with Major Depressive Disorder: Double-Blind Comparison of Nefazodone and Sertraline," *Journal of Clinical Psychiatry* 62 (1): 24–9 (January 2001).

Fieve, Ronald. *Prozac: Questions and Answers for Patients, Family and Physicians.* New York: Avon Books, 1994.

————. *Moodswing.* New York: William Morrow, 1989.

Fink, Max. "Can ECT Be an Effective Treatment for Adolescents?" *Harvard Mental Health Letter* 10 (11): 8 (1994).

Fleming, Jan, and David R. Offord, "Epidemiology of Childhood Depressive Disorders: A Critical Review," *Journal of the American Academy of Child and Adolescent Psychiatry* 29 (4): 571–80 (July 1990).

Frank, Ellen, et al. "Three-Year Outcomes for Maintenance Therapies in Recurrent Depression," *Archives of General Psychiatry* 47 (December 1990): 1093–99.

Frankel, K. A., and R. J. Harmon. "Depressed Mothers: They Don't Always Look as Bad as They Feel," *Journal of the American Academy of Child and Adolescent Psychiatry* 35 (March 1996): 289–98.

Franklin, Deborah. "The Ups and Downs of Prozac," *In Health,* January/February 1991, 24–25.

Freeman, E. W., et al. "A Pilot Study of the Effectiveness of Citalopram in Patients with Premenstrual Syndrome with Prior Selective Serotonin Reuptake Inhibitor Treatment Failure," *Obstetrics and Gynecology* 97 (4) (suppl 1): S18 (April 2001).

Freeman, Hugh. "Meclobemide," *The Lancet* 342 (December 18, 1993): 1528–32.

Freeman, S. J., M. K. Oneil, and W. J. Lance. "Sex Differences in Depression in University Students," *Social Psychiatry* 20 (4): 184–90 (1985).

Gelman, David. "Drugs vs. the Couch," *Newsweek,* March 26, 1990, 42–43.

Glassman, Alexander, et al. "The Safety of Tricyclic Antidepressants in Cardiac Patients: Risk-Benefit Reconsidered," *JAMA* 269 (May 26, 1993): 2673–5.

Goff, D. C., et al. "Trial of Fluoxetine Added to Neuroleptics for Treatment-Resistant Schizophrenic Patients," *American Journal of Psychiatry* 147 (4): 492–4 (April 1990).

Gold, Mark. *The Good News About Depression*. New York: Bantam Books, 1986.

Goodwin, Frederick, and Kay Redfield Jamison. *Manic-Depressive Illness*. New York: Oxford University Press, 1990.

Grady, Denise. "Wonder Drug/Killer Drug: The Furor Over Prozac Won't Go Away," *American Health*, October 1990, 60–65.

Greist, John, and James Jefferson. *Depression and Its Treatment*. New York: Warner Books, 1992.

————. *Dealing with Depression: Taking Steps in the Right Direction*. New York: Pfizer, 1992.

Hadley, A., and M. P. Cason. "Mania Resulting from Lithium-Fluoxetine Combination," letter to author, *American Journal of Psychiatry* 146 (1989): 1637–8.

Hamilton, J. A., B. L. Parry, and S. J. Blumenthal. "The Menstrual Cycle in Context I: Affective Syndromes Associated with Reproductive Hormonal Changes," *Journal of Clinical Psychiatry*, March 1988.

Hanna, M. E., et al. "Severe Lithium Toxicity Associated With Indapamide Therapy," *Journal of Clinical Psychopharmacology* 10 (1990): 379.

Hartter, S., et al. "Differential Effects of Fluvoxamine and Other Antidepressants on the Biotransformation of Melatonin," *Journal of Clinical Psychopharmacology* 21 (2): 167–74 (April 2001).

Harvey, K. V., and R. Balon. "Clinical Implications of Antidepressant Drug Effects on Sexual Function," *Annals of Clinical Psychiatry* 7 (December 1995): 189–201.

Hellerstein, D. J., et al. "A Randomized Double-Blind Study of Fluoxetine Versus Placebo in the Treatment of Dysthymia," *American Journal of Psychiatry* 150 (8): 1169–1975 (1993).

Herman, John B., et al. "Fluoxetine-Induced Sexual Dysfunction," *Journal of Clinical Psychiatry* 51 (January 1990): 25–27.

"High Anxiety," *Consumer Reports* 58 (January 1993): 19–24.

Higley, J. Dee, et al. "Cerebrospinal Fluid Monoamine and Adrenal Correlates of Aggression in Free-Ranging Rhesus Monkeys," *Archives of General Psychiatry* 49 (6): 436–41 (June 1992).

Hirschfield, R. M. A., et al. "The National Depressive and Manic-Depressive Association Consensus Statement on the Undertreatment of Depression," *JAMA* 277 (January 22–29, 1997): 333–40.

Hochstrasser, B., et. al. "Prophylactic Effect of Citalopram in Unipolar, Recurrent Depression: Placebo-Controlled Study of Maintenance Therapy," *British Journal of Psychiatry* 178 (4): 304–10 (April 2001).

Holden, C. "Depression: The News Isn't Depressing," *Science* 254 (1991): 1450–2.

Hollander, Eric, and Allison McCarley. "Yohimbine Treatment of Sexual Side Effects Induced by Serotonin Reuptake Blockers," *Journal of Clinical Psychiatry* 53 (1992): 207–9.

Hoover, C. E. "Suicidal Ideation Not Associated with Fluoxetine," letter to author, *American Journal of Psychiatry* 148 (1991): 543.

Jefferson, James, and John Greist. *Depression and Adolescents: Recognizing the Signs of Depression and Taking Steps to Help.* New York: Pfizer, 1993.

———. *Depression and Older People: Recognizing Hidden Signs and Taking Steps Toward Recovery.* New York: Pfizer, 1993.

Jerome, L. "Hypomania with Fluoxetine," *Journal of American Academy of Child and Adolescent Psychiatry* 30 (5): 850–1 (1991).

Joffe, et al. "Clinical Features of Situational and Nonsituational Major Depression," *Psychopathology* 26 (3–4): 138–44 (1993).

Jonas, Jeffrey, and Ron Schaumburg. *Everything You Need to Know About Prozac.* New York: Bantam Books, 1991.

Kapur, Shitij, et al. "Antidepressant Medications and the Relative Risk of Suicide Attempt and Suicide," *JAMA* 268 (December 23, 1992): 3441–5.

Karasu, T. Byrum. "Toward a Clinical Model of Psychotherapy for Depression II: An Integrative and Selective Treatment Approach," *American Journal of Psychiatry* 147 (March 1990): 269–78.

Kendler, K. S. "Risk Factors in the Familial Aggregation of Psychiatric Disorders," *Psychosomatic Medicine* 20 (2): 311–19 (1990).

Kendler, K. S., et al. "Major Depression and Generalized Anxiety Disorder: Same Genes, (Partly) Different Environments?" *Archives of General Psychiatry* 49 (1992): 716–22.

Klein, D. F., and P. H. Wender. *Understanding Depression: A Complete Guide to Its Diagnosis and Treatment.* New York: Oxford University Press, 1993.

Klerman, G. L., and M. M. Weisman. "Increasing Rates of Depression," *JAMA* 261 (1989): 2229–35.

Konig, F., et al. "First Experiences in Combination Therapy Using Olanzapine with SSRIs (Citalopram, Paroxetine) in Delusional Depression," *Neuropsychobiology* 43 (3): 170–74 (March 2001).

Koren, G. "First Trimester Exposure to Fluoxetine (Prozac). Does It Affect Pregnancy Outcome?" *Canadian Family Physician* 42 (January 1996): 43–4.

Kramer, Peter. *Listening to Prozac.* New York: Viking Press, 1993.

Kupfer, David J. "Long-Term Treatment of Depression," *Journal of Clinical Psychiatry* 52 (5): 28–34 (May 1991).

Larkin, Ellen. "Depression and Advancing Age," *FDA Consumer* 27 (March 1993): 18–22.

Leibenluft, E. "Women with Bipolar Illness: Clinical and Research Issues," *American Journal of Psychiatry* 153 (February 1996): 163–73.

Liebowitz, M. R., et al. "Fluoxetine for Adolescents with Obsessive-Compulsive Disorder," *American Journal of Psychiatry* 147 (3): 370–1 (March 1990).

"Lifetime and Twelve-Month Prevalence of DSM-III-R Psychiatric Disorders in the United States," *Archives of General Psychiatry* 51 (January 1994): 8–19.

Linde, Klaus, et al. "St. John's Wort for Depression—An Overview and Metaanalysis of Randomised Clinical Trials," *British Medical Journal* 313 (1996): 253–8.

Long, James. *Essential Guide to Prescription Drugs.* New York: HarperCollins, 1994.

Maj, Mario, et al. "Pattern of Recurrence of Illness After Recovery from an Episode of Major Depression: A Prospective Study," *American Journal of Psychiatry* 149 (June 1992): 795–800.

Mann, J. J., et al. "Relationship Between Central and Peripheral Serotonin Indexes in Depressed and Suicidal Psychiatric Inpatients," *Archives of General Psychiatry* 49 (6): 442–59 (June 1992).

Mann, J. J., and S. Kapur. "The Emergence of Suicidal Ideation and Behavior During Antidepressant Therapy," *Archives of General Psychiatry* 48 (November 1991): 1027–33.

Manos, G. H. "Possible Serotonin Syndrome Associated with Buspirone Added to Fluoxetine," *Annals of Pharmacotherapy* 34 (7–8): 871–4 (July/August 2000).

Marcus, M. D., et al. "A Double-Blind, Placebo-Controlled Trial of Fluoxetine Plus Behavior Modification in the Treatment of Obese Binge-Eaters and Non-Binge-Eaters," *American Journal of Psychiatry* 147 (7): 876–81 (July 1990).

Markovitz, P. J., S. J. Stagno, and J. R. Calabrese. "Buspirone Augmentation of Fluoxetine in Obsessive-Compulsive Disorder," *American Journal of Psychiatry* 147 (6): 798–800 (June 1990).

Marx, Jean. "Do Antidepressants Promote Tumors?" *Science* 257 (July 3, 1992): 22–23.

McEnay, Geoffrey. "Nursing the Mind: Managing Mood Disorders," *RN* 53 (September 1990): 28–33.

McGrath, Ellen. *When Feeling Bad Is Good*. New York: Bantam Books, 1994.

Michael, A., and E. A. O'Donnell. "Fluoxetine-Induced Sexual Dysfunction Reversed by Trazodone," *Canadian Journal of Psychiatry* 45 (9): 847–8 (November 2000).

Milani, R. V., et al. "Effects of Cardiac Rehabilitation and Exercise Training Programs on Depression in Patients After Major Coronary Events," *American Heart Journal* 132 (October 1996): 726–32.

Mitka, Mike. "Drug Maker to Defend Physicians Sued over Prozac," *American Medical News* 34 (June 24, 1991): 14.

Mohan, C. G., and J. J. Moore. "Fluoxetine Toxicity in a Preterm Infant," *Journal of Perinatology* 20 (7): 445–6 (October/November 2000).

Moore, Jeffrey, and Robert Rodriguez. "Toxicity of Fluoxetine in Overdose," *American Journal of Psychiatry* 147 (August 1990): 1089.

Mulcahey, J. J., et al. "Serotonin-Selective Reuptake Inhibitors in the Treatment of Geriatric Depression and Related Disorders," *International Journal of Neuropsychopharmcology* 2 (2): 121–7 (June 1999).

Munoz, Ricardo, et al. "On the AHCPR Depression in Primary Care Guidelines," *American Psychologist* 49 (1): 42–61 (January 1994).

Musa, M. N., and J. M. Staneluis. "Adverse Events of Fluoxetine: Postmarketing Compared with Premarketing Clinical Trials," *Journal of Clinical Psychiatry* 61 (11): 874 (November 2000).

Musselman, D. L., et al. "Paroxetine for the Prevention of Depression Induced by High-Dose Interferon Alfa," *New England Journal of Medicine* 344 (13): 961–6 (March 29, 2001).

Nakra, B. R., et al. "Mania Induced by Fluoxetine," letter to author, *American Journal of Psychiatry* 146 (11): 1515–16 (November 1989).

Narurkar, Vic. "Desipramine-Induced Blue-Gray Photosensitive Pigmentation," *JAMA* 270 (July 7, 1993): 28.

Nemeroff, Charles B., et al. "Adrenal Gland Enlargement in Major Depression: A Computed Tomographic Study," *Archives of General Psychiatry* 49 (May 1992): 384–87.

Neziroglu, F., et al. "The Effect of Fluvoxamine and Behavior Therapy on Children and Adolescents with Obsessive-Compulsive Disorder," *Journal of Child and Adolescent Psychopharmacology* 10 (4): 295–306 (winter 2000).

1994 Physician's Desk Reference. Montvale, N.J.: Medical Economics Data Production Co., 1994.

Ni, Y. G., and R. Miledi. "Blockage of 5HT2C Serotonin Receptors by Fluoxetine (Prozac)," *Proceeds of the National Academy of Science USA* 94 (March 4, 1997): 2036–40.

Nolen-Hoeksema, Susan. *Sex Differences in Depression.* Stanford, Calif.: Stanford University Press, 1990.

Nulman, Irena, et al. "Neurodevelopment of Children Exposed in Utero to Antidepressant Drugs," *New England Journal of Medicine* 336 (1997): 258–62.

Nussar, Daniel. *Modell's Drugs in Current Use and New Drugs.* New York: Springer Publishing, 1993.

Ornstein, Robert, and C. Swencionis. *The Healing Brain: A Scientific Reader.* New York: Guilford Press, 1990.

Panzarino, P. J., Jr., and D. B. Nash. "Cost-Effective Treatment of Depression with Selective Serotonin Reuptake Inhibitors," *American Journal of Managed Care* 7 (2): 173–84 (February 2001).

Papolos, Demitri, and Janice Papolos. *Overcoming Depression.* New York: Harper Press, 1992.

Papp, L., and J. Gorman. "Suicidal Preoccupation During Fluoxetine Treatment," letter to author, *American Journal of Psychiatry* 147 (10): 1380–1 (October 1990).

Paradis, Cynthia. "Nortriptyline and Weight Change in Depressed Patients Over 60," *JAMA* 269 (January 6, 1993): 99.

Pastuszak, Anne, et al. "Pregnancy Outcome Following First-Trimester Exposure to Fluoxetine (Prozac)," *JAMA* 269 (May 5, 1993): 2246–8.

Perino, C., et al. "Mood and Behavioral Disorders Following Traumatic Brain Injury: Clinical Evaluation and Pharmacological Management," *Brain Injury* 15 (2): 139–48 (February 2001).

Peterson, M. C. "Reversible Galactorrhea and Prolactin Elevation Related to Fluoxetine Use," *Mayo Clinic Proceedings* 76·(2): 215–16 (February 2001).

Pettinati, H. M., et al. "Double-Blind Clinical Trial of Sertraline Treatment for Alcohol Dependence," *Journal of Clinical Psychopharmacology* 21 (2): 143–53 (April 2001).

Pharmaceutical Research and Manufacturers of America. "In Development: New Medicines for Mental Illness," *New Medicines in Development Series,* Washington, D.C.: May 1994.

Pigott, T. A., et al. "Controlled Comparisons of Clomipramine and Fluoxetine in the Treatment of Obsessive-Compulsive Disorder: Behavioral and Biological Results," *Archives of General Psychiatry* 48 (9): 857–9 (September 1991).

Piredda, S. G., and S. L. Rubinstein. "Hypomania Induced by Fluoxetine," *Biological Psychiatry* 32 (1): 107 (July 1, 1992).

Pollack, M. H., et al. "Sertraline Treatment of Panic Disorder: Response in Patients at Risk for Poor Outcome," *Journal of Clinical Psychiatry* 61 (12): 922–7 (December 2000).

————, and J. F. Rosenbaum. "Fluoxetine Treatment of Cocaine Abuse in Heroin Addicts," *Journal of Clinical Psychiatry* 52 (1): 31–33 (January 1991).

Post, Robert M., and James C. Ballenger. "Sensitization and Kindling Perspectives for the Course of Affective Illness: Toward a New Treatment with the Anticonvulsant Carbamazepine," *Pharmacopsychiatry* 23 (1990): 3–17.

————, et al. "Carbamazepine Prophylaxis in Refractory Affective Disorders: A Focus on Long-Term Follow-Up," *Journal of Clinical Psychopharmacology* 10 (1990): 318–27.

Potter, William. "The Pharmacologic Treatment of Depression," *The New England Journal of Medicine* 325 (August 29, 1991): 633–42.

Preskorn, S. H., and M. Burke. "Somatic Therapy for Major Depressive Disorder: Selection of an Antidepressant," *Journal of Clinical Psychiatry* 53 (9) (suppl): 5–18 (1992).

————, et al. "Serious Adverse Effects of Combining Fluoxetine and Tricyclic Antidepressants," letter to author, *American Journal of Psychiatry* 147 (4): 532 (April 1990).

Prien, Robert F., and Alan J. Gelenberg. "Alternatives to Lithium for Preventive Treatment of Bipolar Disorder," *American Journal of Psychiatry* 146 (1990): 840–8.

Rakel, Robert, ed. *Conn's Current Therapy.* Philadelphia: W. B. Saunders, 1993.

Ramirez, L. C., et al. "Effective Treatment of Bulimia with Fluoxetine, a Serotonin Uptake Inhibitor in a Patient with Type 1 Diabetes Mellitus," *The American Journal of Medicine* 88 (May 1990): 540–1.

Reaves, John, and James B. Austin. *How to Find Help for a Troubled Kid: A Parent's Guide to Programs and Services for Adolescents.* New York: Henry Holt, 1990.

Reynolds, C. F. "Treatment of Depression in Special Populations," *Journal of Clinical Psychiatry* 53 (9): 45–53 (1992).

Rinzler, Carol Ann. *Are You at Risk?* New York: Facts on File, 1991.

Romano, S., et al. "Long-Term Treatment of Obsessive-Compulsive Disorder After an Acute Response: A Comparison of Fluoxetine versus Placebo," *Journal of Clinical Psychopharmacology* 21 (1): 46–52 (February 2001).

Rosenfeld, Isadore. *The Best Treatment.* New York: Simon & Schuster, 1991.

Rosenthal, Norman E. *Seasons of the Mind.* New York: Bantam Books, 1990.

Rudolph, R., and A. D. Feiger. "A Double-Blind, Randomized, Placebo-Controlled Trial of Once-Daily Venlafaxine Extended Release (XR) and Fluoxetine for the Treatment of Depression," *Journal of Affective Disorders* 56 (2–3): 171–81 (December 1999).

Rush, A. J. "Problems Associated with Diagnosis of Depression," *Journal of Clinical Psychiatry* 51 (6): 15–22 (1990).

Sacra, Cheryl. "The New Cure-Alls: Mood Lifters May Offer Handfuls of Hope for More Than Just Depression," *Health,* September 1990, 36–8.

Saline, Carol. "Don't Blame Prozac," *Philadelphia Magazine,* August 1991, 49–53.

Schad-Somers, Susanne P. *On Mood Swings: The Psychobiology of Elation and Depression.* New York: Plenum Press, 1990.

Schatzberg, A. F. "Dosing Strategies for Antidepressant Agents," *Journal of Clinical Psychiatry* 52 (5) (suppl): 14–20 (1991).

————, and J. O. Cole. *Manual of Clinical Psychopharmacology*. 2d ed. Washington, D.C.: American Psychiatric Press, 1991.

Schmidt, M. E., et al. "The Efficacy and Safety of a New Enteric-Coated Formulation of Fluoxetine Given Once Weekly During the Continuation Treatment of Major Depressive Disorder," *Journal of Clinical Psychiatry* 61 (11): 851–7 (November 2000).

Schneier, F. R. "Treatment of Social Phobia with Antidepressants," *Journal of Clinical Psychiatry* 62 (suppl) (1): 43–8, discussion 49 (2001).

————, et al. "Fluoxetine in Panic Disorders," *Journal of Clinical Psychopharmacology* 10 (2): 119–21 (1990).

Schuchman, Miriam, and Michael Wilkes. "Dramatic Progress Against Depression," *The New York Times Magazine*, October 7, 1990, S12.

Schulkin, Jay. "Melancholic Depression and the Hormones of Adversity: A Role for the Amygdala," *Current Directions in Psychological Science* 3 (2): 41–4 (April 1994).

Schumer, Fran. "Bye-Bye, Blues: A New Wonder Drug for Depression," *New York*, December 18, 1989, 48–53.

Schwartz, John. "The Drug Did It: A Tough Sell in Court," *Newsweek*, April 1, 1991, 66.

"Scientology: The Cult of Greed," *Time*, May 6, 1991, 32–39.

Seligman, Martin. *Learned Optimism*. New York: Alfred Knopf, 1991.

Shapiro, Patricia Gottleib. *A Parents' Guide to Childhood and Adolescent Depression*. New York: Dell Publishing, 1994.

Simpson, S. G., and J. R. DePaulo. "Fluoxetine Treatment of Bipolar II Depression," *Journal of Clinical Psychopharmacology* 11 (1): 52–54 (1991).

Skelly, Flora Johnson. "The Hype About Prozac: Here's How to Answer Your Patients' Questions and Improve Your Treatment of Chronic Depression," *American Medical News* 36 (December 6, 1993): 13–15.

Slap, Gail, et al. "Risk Factors for Attempted Suicide During Adolescence," *Pediatrics* 84 (5): 769 (November 1989).

Sleek, Scott. "Could Prozac Replace Demand for Therapy?" *APA Monitor*, April 1994, 28.

Snyder, Solomon. *The New Biology of Mood*. New York: Pfizer, 1988.

Stanford, S. C. "Prozac: Panacea or Puzzle?" *Trends in Pharmacological Science* 17 (April 1996): 150–4.

Stein, Dan J., et al. "Serotonergic Medications for Sexual Obsessions, Sexual Addictions and Paraphilias," *Journal of Clinical Psychiatry* 53 (1992): 267–71.

Sternbach, H. "The Serotonin Syndrome," *American Journal of Psychiatry* 148 (1991): 705–13.

Stinson, Stephen. "Psychoactive Drugs," *Chemical & Engineering News* 68 (October 15, 1990): 33–50.

Stokes, P. "The Changing Horizon in the Treatment of Depression: Scientific/Clinical Publication Overview," *Journal of Clinical Psychiatry* 52 (5): 35–43 (1991).

Styron, William. *Darkness Visible: A Memoir of Madness*. New York: Random House, 1990.

Suri, R. A., et al. "Efficacy and Response Time to Sertraline versus Fluoxetine in the Treatment of Unipolar Major Depressive Disorder," *Journal of Clinical Psychiatry* 61 (12): 942–6 (December 2000).

"Tailoring Treatment for Depression's Many Forms," *U.S. News & World Report*, March 5, 1990, 54–5.

Teicher, Martin, et al. "Emergence of Intense Suicidal Preoccupation During Fluoxetine Treatment," *American Journal of Psychiatry* 147 (February 1990): 207–10.

Thomas, Patricia. "Sad Attack," *Harvard Health Letter*, October 1991, 1–4.

Thornton, Jim. "Pharm Aid: Ten New Medicines You Should Know About," *Men's Health,* October 1990, 73–77.

Toufexis, Anastasia. "The Personality Pill," *Time,* October 11, 1993, 61–2.

———. "Warnings About a Miracle Drug: Reports of Suicide Attempts in Prozac Users Raise Doubts About the Popular Antidepressant," *Time,* July 30, 1990, 54.

Turkington, Carol A. *The Hypericum Handbook.* New York: Barnes & Noble Books, 1998.

"Uplifting Pill," *Discover,* June 1991, 14–5.

U.S. Department of Health and Human Services. *Special Report on Depression Research,* Rockville, Md.: 1983.

Venkataraman, S., et al. "Mania Associated with Fluoxetine Treatment in Adolescents," *Journal of the American Academy of Child and Adolescent Psychiatry* 31 (2): 276–81 (1992).

Wade, G. S. "Controlled Withdrawal for Psychotropic Drugs," *The Lancet* 355 (9217): 1822–3 (May 20, 2000).

Wartik, Nancy. "Depression: An Array of New Treatments Combats the Common Cold of Mental Illness," and "Manic-Depression: Not for Artists Only," *American Health,* December 1993, 39–42.

Wehr, T. A., and F. K. Goodwin. "Can Antidepressants Cause Mania and Worsen the Course of Affective Illness?" *American Journal of Psychiatry* 144 (11): 1403–11 (1987).

Weintraub, Pamela. "Warning: Side Effects," *American Health,* April 1992, 36–7.

Wells, K. B., et al. "The Functioning and Well-Being of Depressed Patients: Results from the Medical Outcomes Study," *JAMA* 262 (1989): 914–19.

Willensky, Diana. "Once in a Blue Mood," *American Health,* April 1991, 12.

Winokur, George, et al. "Familial Alcoholism in Manic-Depressive (Bipolar) Disease," *American Journal of Medical Genetics* 67 (April 9, 1996): 197–201.

————, et al. "Further Distinctions Between Manic-Depressive Illness (Bipolar Disorder) and Primary Depressive Disorder (Unipolar Depression)," *American Journal of Psychiatry* 150 (8): 1176–81 (August 1993).

Wirshing, W. C., et al. "Fluoxetine, Akathisia and Suicidality: Is There a Causal Connection?" letter to author, *Archives of General Psychiatry* 49: 580–1 (1992).

Wise, M. G., and S. E. Taylor. "Anxiety and Mood Disorders in Medically Ill Patients," *Journal of Clinical Psychiatry* 51 (1): 27–32 (1990).

"Worried About Prozac," *Consumer Reports* 58 (October 1993): 636.

Zajecka, John, et al. "The Role of Serotonin in Sexual Dysfunction: Fluoxetine-Associated Orgasm Dysfunction," *Journal of Clinical Psychiatry* 52 (2): 66–8 (February 1991).

ORGANIZATIONS

Agency for Health Care Policy and Research
   Executive Office Center
   2101 East Jefferson St., Suite 501
   Rockville, MD 20852
   (800) 255-1708
   (301) 594-1364
   www.ahcpr.gov
   (Provides general information on depression)

American Academy of Child and Adolescent Psychiatry
   3615 Wisconsin Ave. NW
   Washington, DC 20016
   (202) 966-7300
   www.aacap.org
   (Publishes free written material including "Facts
   for Families": 45 fact sheets covering issues of
   normal childhood and disorders)

Anxiety Disorders Association of America
   11900 Parklawn Dr., Suite 100
   Rockville, MD 20852
   (301) 231-9350
   www.adaa.org

D/ART Program
(Depression/Awareness, Recognition, and Treatment)
National Institute of Mental Health
5600 Fishers Lane
Room 10C-03
Bethesda, MD 20892
(800) 421-4211
(Provides free brochures about depression)

Depressed Anonymous
PO Box 17414
Louisville, KY 40217
(502) 459-6700
www.depressedanon.com
(12-step program with newsletter, phone support, information and referrals, pen pals, workshops, conferences, and seminars. Information pack $5; D.A. manual $12)

Depression and Related Affective Disorders Association
Meyer 3-181
600 N. Wolfe St.
Baltimore, MD 21287
(410) 955-4647
www.med.jhu.edu/drada
(Provides education and information and supporting research, with newsletter, literature, phone support; offers Young People's Outreach Project and Depression in the Workplace Project)

Depression After Delivery
PO Box 278
Belle Mead, PA 08502
(908) 575-9121
(800) 944-4773 (to leave name and address for
information to be sent)
www.behavenet.com/dadinc
(Provides support and information for women
who have postpartum depression, with telephone
support in most states, newsletter [$30/year],
group development guidelines, pen pals, and
conferences)

Emotions Anonymous
PO Box 4245
St. Paul, MN 55104
(651) 647-9712
www.emotionsanonymous.org
(Telephone referrals to local chapters; publications
available)

Federation of Families for Children's Mental Health
1101 King St.
Alexandria, VA 22314
(703) 684-7710
www.ffcmh.org
(Parent-run volunteer group makes referrals
to professionals and other parents throughout
America)

National Alliance for the Mentally Ill
    Colonial Place Three
    2107 Wilson Blvd., Suite 300
    Arlington, VA 22201
    (703) 524-7600
    (800) 950-NAMI (6264)
    www.nami.org
    (Provides support groups for the families of the
    mentally ill; call the 800-number for location of a
    local group in your area)

National Depressive and Manic-Depressive Association
    730 North Franklin St., Suite 501
    Chicago, IL 60610
    (312) 642-0049
    (800) 826-3632
    (312) 642-7243 (FAX)
    www.ndmda.org
    (Offers information on depression and manic-
    depression, one-on-one support, referrals by
    phone; publications and audiotapes and videotapes;
    to locate a depressed-patient support group, call the
    800-number between 8:30 A.M. and 5 P.M. CST)

National Foundation for Depressive Illness
    PO Box 2257
    New York, NY 10116
    (212) 268-4260
    Hotline: (800) 239-1265
    www.depression.org
    (Recorded information about the symptoms
    and treatment of depression, how to obtain

an information packet with a list of doctors who specialize in treating depression, and support groups in your area)

National Institute of Mental Health
Public Inquiries
6001 Executive Blvd.
Room 8184, MSC 9663
Bethesda, MD 20892
(301) 443-4513
www.nimh.nih.gov
(For a free copy of *Depression Is a Treatable Illness*, send a postcard asking for the "Depression Guide" to the above address)

National Mental Health Association
1021 Prince St.
Alexandria, VA 22314
(800) 969-6642
(703) 684-7722
www.nmha.org
(Helpful publications on depression, list of local chapters for referral to support groups, home-based services, and professionals in your area)

National Organization for Seasonal Affective Disorder (NOSAD)
PO Box 40133
Washington, DC 20016
www.nosad.org
(Newsletter, support groups, information about SAD)

Obsessive-Compulsive Foundation, Inc.
337 Notch Hill Rd.
N. Branford, CT 06471
(203) 315-2190
www.ocfoundation.org

Postpartum Support International
927 N. Kellog Ave.
Santa Barbara, CA 93111
(805) 967-7636 (daytime PST)
www.chss.iup.edu/postpartum
(Provides education, advocacy, annual conference,
encourages formation of support groups, phone
support, referrals, literature, and newsletter)

Recovery, Inc.
802 N. Dearborn St.
Chicago, IL 60610
(312) 337-5661
www.recovery-inc.com
(A community mental health organization that
offers a self-help method of will training with a
method of techniques for controlling behavior and
changing attitudes toward nervous symptoms,
anxiety, depression, anger, and fear; publishes
"Recovery Reporter" for members; provides
information on starting groups and leadership
training)

Research and Training Center on Family Support and
Children's Mental Health
  Regional Research Institute
  Portland State University
  PO Box 751
  Portland, OR 97207
  (503) 725-4040
  www.rtc.pdx.edu
  (Maintains computerized database covering profes-
  sionals, organizations, and parent groups all over the
  United States; distributes literature on depression
  and other issues related to children's mental health)

Society for Light Treatment and Biological Rhythms
  PO Box 591687
  174 Cook St.
  San Francisco, CA 94159
  www.sltbr.org
  (Provides further information on seasonal affective
  depression and light therapy)

How to Find Names of Local Mental-Health Professionals

Psychiatrists

American Academy of Child and Adolescent Psychiatry
3615 Wisconsin Ave. NW
Washington, DC 20016
(202) 966-2891
www.aacap.org
(References to child and adolescent psychiatrists in local areas)

American Psychiatric Association
1400 K St. NW
Washington, DC 20005
(888) 357-7924
www.psych.org
(Provides telephone numbers of district branches, which will refer to psychiatrist specialists in your area)

Psychologists

American Psychological Association
750 First Ave. NE
Washington, DC 20002-2424
(202) 336-5700
www.apa.org
(Provides phone number of your state organization,
which will make referrals to psychologists in your area)

APPENDIX C

TWELVE-STEP PROGRAMS

All sorts of substances may be abused by depressed people trying to numb specific symptoms. Unfortunately, drugs and alcohol generally only worsen depression. Following is a list of self-help programs based on the well-known "12-step" method popularized by Alcoholics Anonymous.

Alcoholics Anonymous
 475 Riverside Dr., 11th floor
 PO Box 459
 Grand Central Station
 New York, NY 10163
 (212) 870-3400
 www.alcoholics-anonymous.org

Al-Anon Family Groups Headquarters, Inc.
 1600 Corporate Landing Parkway
 Virginia Beach, VA 23454
 (800) 344-2666
 www.al-anon.alateen.org

A.R.T.S. Anonymous (Artists Recovering Through the Twelve Steps)
 PO Box 230175
 New York, NY 10023
 (212) 873-7075

Cocaine Anonymous
    3740 Overland Ave., Suite C
    Los Angeles, CA 90034
    (310) 559-5833
    www.ca.org

CoDependents Anonymous
    PO Box 33577
    Phoenix, AZ 85067
    (602) 277-7991 (in New York: [212] 691-5199)
    www.codependents.org

Emotions Anonymous
    PO Box 4245
    St. Paul, MN 55104
    (651) 647-9712
    www.emotionsanonymous.org

Gamblers Anonymous
    PO Box 17173
    Los Angeles, CA 90017
    (213) 386-8789
    www.gamblersanonymous.org

Narcotics Anonymous
    16155 Wyandotte St.
    PO Box 9999
    Van Nuys, CA 91409
    (818) 773-9999
    www.na.org

Nicotine Anonymous
    419 Main St., PMB 370
    Huntington Beach, CA 92648
    (866) 536-4539
    www.nicotine-anonymous.org

Overeaters Anonymous
    6075 Zenith Ct. NE
    Rio Rancho, NM 87124
    (505) 891-2664
    www.overeatersanonymous.org

Sex Addicts Anonymous
    PO Box 70949
    Houston, TX 77270
    (800) 477-8191
    (713) 869-4902
    www.sexaa.org

Workaholics Anonymous
    PO Box 289
    Menlo Park, CA 94026
    (510) 273-9253

Depression Links on the World Wide Web

Antidepressants

Antidepressant Information
A site that gives detailed information on any drug name, together with its chemical formula and other technical information about dosage, side effects, and precautions. Search by brand name, manufacturer, or generic name.
www.druginfonet.com/index.html

Internet Mental Health: Drugs
A relatively technical path that explains antidepressants, including the symptoms they are used to treat, how the drugs work, when they shouldn't be used, and warnings and guidelines for pregnancy, geriatrics, and drug inter-actions. The site also includes symptoms of overdose, dosage instructions, and the exact contents of the pill or liquid.
www.mentalhealth.com/fr30.html

Rx List
Yet another source for drug information. Type in the name of any drug (brand or generic) and you'll receive a list of symptoms it's designed to treat, side effects, adverse reactions, and other information on related drugs.
www.rxlist.com

Bipolar Disorder (Manic-Depression)

Bipolar Disorder
Diagnostic criteria, treatments, suicide, news articles, lists of books and movies, and tips for tracing bipolar illness in your family.
www.frii.com/~parrot/bip.html

Moodswing.org
The new home of the Bipolar Diorder FAQ, with a database of support groups, clinics, physicians, and psychologists who deal with manic-depression. A bipolar disorder message board and a regularly scheduled chat session are available, together with an online catalog of some of the most recommended books dealing with bipolar disorder.
www.moodswing.org/

Depression
Informative site discussing depression in teens, the elderly, and those with chronic illness; packed with all sorts of information and links on origin, treatment, types of depression, weight and depression, suicide, and more.
www.depression.org

Depression—Children/Adolescents

Depression in Children
Information to help educate parents and families about psychiatric disorders affecting children and adolescents.
www.nimh.nih.gov/publicat/depchildresfact.cfm

Manic-Depression in Teens
Information to help educate parents and families about
teens and bipolar disorder.
www.windsofchange.com

Teenage Depression
Frequently asked questions about the rise of depression
during teenage years, with information to help detect suicide risk.
www.mentalhealth.com/mag1/p51-dp01.html

Depression—General

Suicide and Suicide Prevention
Information on suicide, serotonin, statistics, depression,
and much more.
www.psycom.net/depression.central.suicide.html

Depression and Mental Health
An index of links with one-word descriptions that includes
information such as symptoms of depression and questions
and answers about depression.
drycas.club.cc.cmu.edu/~maire/depress.html

Depression Central
A page of links to depression, mood, and related disorders
resources online maintained by a long-standing Internet
psychiatrist Ivan Goldberg. You'll find lots of research and
professional articles usually not included elsewhere.
www.psycom.net/depression.central.html

Depression Home Page
Resources divided into the areas of education, commercial, and miscellaneous.
www.isca.uiowa.edu/users/david-caropreso/depression.html

Mood Disorders
Information on a wide variety of problems from depression to seasonal affective disorder, with access to the depression FAQ (including information on causes, treatment, and medication with a depression primer outlining basic definitions and concepts). Other materials include articles on Prozac and other specific drugs.
www.avocado.pc.helsinki.fi/~janne/mood/mood.html

National Institutes of Mental Health
Informational Brochures
Online access to brochures on bipolar disorder, facts about depressive illnesses, geriatric depression, suicide fact sheet, general information about depression, and suicide journal references.
www.nimh.nih.gov/publicat/bipolar.html

National Library of Medicine (Gopher)
Information on depression and consumer information and how to screen for depression.
gopher://gopher.nim.nih.gov:70/11/hstat/ahcpr/depress/TEMPgrp3

Overcoming Depression and Preventing Suicide
(State University of New York/Buffalo)
General information about depression including symptoms; this site includes the alt.support.depression FAQ.
wings.buffalo.edu/student-life/ccenter/Depression/

Pendulum Resources
Comprehensive information source for bipolar disorder and other mood disorders, including articles, online support groups, and more.
www.pendulum.org/

Internet Depression Resources
A large listing of online depression resources as well as links to personal stories of dealing with depression.
www.geocities.com/HotSprings/8376/

Mental Health Sources on the Internet
Another list of resources, including the Beck Depression Inventory and the best and worst things to say to someone who is depressed.
stripe.Colorado.EDU/~judy/depression/

Suicide Helpline
Links to helpful mailing lists and common suicidal resources online.
www.coil.com/~grohol/helpme.htm

Depression Screening Tests

Clinical Depression Screening Test
This checklist can help determine if you or someone you know is suffering from depression; results are given online.
sandbox.xerox.com/pair/cw/testing.html

Online Screening Test (NYU Psychiatry Department)
Interactive quick screening test with online results designed to give a preliminary idea about the presence of mild to moderate depressive symptoms that indicate the need for an evaluation by a mental health professional.
www.med.nyu.edu/Psych/screens/depres.html

Depression—Seasonal Affective Depression

SAD
This website presents the facts on Seasonal Affective Depression from a clinic in Cambridge, England, together with information on symptoms and treatments, a product catalog, and research abstracts.
www.outsidein.co.uk/bodyclock/sadinfo.html

Seasonal Affective Disorder
(University of British Columbia)
Maintained by a branch of the university's psychiatry project, this site provides information on symptoms, treatments, and suggested readings for SAD.
www.psychiatry.ubc.ca/mood/md_sad.html

Suicide

Suicide: Read This First
Conversations and writings for suicidal persons, with a few simple prevention materials and links to other helpful sites.
www.geocities.com/RainForest/1801/suicide1.html

Suicide Prevention
This website for the Suicide Awareness, Voices of Education (SAVE) organization offers detailed information about identifying, treating, and stablilizing depression to avoid suicide, common statistics, symptoms of depression, a book list, and more.
www.save.org

Suicide Counseling Via E-mail
For anyone contemplating suicide, the Samaritans (a 40-year-old counseling group in the United Kingdom) provides service via E-mail. Trained volunteers answer requests for information using the name "Jo." Those requesting information will receive the FAQ file containing directions about anonymously E-mailing the Samaritans.
E-mail: jo@samaritans.org

Suicide FAQ
This FAQ addresses common problems in caring for a depressed friend or family member.
www.lib.ox.ac.uk/internet/news/faq/archive/ suicide.info.html

Bipolar Disorder
Symptoms, treatment, resources, and much more on this
Mental Health Net site.
bipolar.mentalhelp.net

Suicide Prevention
A brochure that tries to help identify those at risk for suicide, listing danger signals (including words and actions
to watch for), and facts and statistics that dispel some
myths about suicide.
www.odos.uiuc.edu/Counseling_Center/suiprev.html

Newsgroups

alt.support.depression (depression and mood disorders)
alt.support.depression.manic (manic-depression and
    bipolar disorders)
alt.support.depression.seasonal (seasonal affective
    disorder, or SAD)
sci.med.psychobiology (dialogue and news in psychiatry
    and psychobiology)
sci.psychology.misc (general discussion of psychology)
sci.psychology.psychotherapy (practice of psychotherapy)
soc.support.depression.crisis (personal crisis situations)
soc.support.depression.family (coping with depressed
    people)
soc.support.depression.manic (bipolar, manic-depression)
soc.support.depression.misc (depression and mood
    disorders)

soc.support.depression.seasonal (seasonal affective disorder, or SAD)

soc.support.depression.treatment (treatments of depression)

Mailing Lists

bipolar disorder (manic-depression)
majordomo@ucar.edu

depression and bipolar disorder
walkers-request@world.std.com

depression, Christian-oriented
hub@xc.org

partners and family of depressed people
majordomo@truespectra.com

suicide support
suicide-support-request@research.canon.com.au

suicide survivors
suicide-survivors-request@research.canon.com.au

Free Medication Programs for Low-Income Patients

Some drug companies offer free medication to low-income families. They require a doctor's consent and proof of financial status—but in some cases, a few companies allow family incomes as high as $40,000 a year if it's offset by enough expenses. *Note: Some of these companies may prefer to speak directly to your doctor.*

BuSpar
Bristol-Myers Squibb
Company
(800) 332-2056

Depakote
Abbott Labs
(800) 441-4987

Desyrel
(150 and 300 milligram
pills only)
Bristol-Myers Squibb
Company
(800) 332-2056

Effexor
Wyeth-Ayerst Laboratories
(703) 706-5933

Elavil
Zeneca Pharmaceuticals
(800) 424-3727

Ludiomil
Lederle Laboratories
(703) 706-5933

Luvox
Solvay Pharmaceuticals, Inc.
(218) 634-3500

Norpramin
Hoechst Marion Roussel,
Inc.
(800) 221-4025

Parnate
Scios, Inc.
(800) 633-0711

Paxil
SmithKline Beecham
Pharmaceuticals
(800) 546-0420

Prozac
Eli Lilly & Co.
(800) 545-6962

Remeron
Organon
(800) 241-8812

Serzone
Bristol-Myers Squibb
Company
(800) 332-2056

Surmontil
Wyeth-Ayerst Laboratories
(703) 706-5933

Tegretol
Novartis Pharmaceuticals
(800) 257-3273

Valium
Roche Laboratories, Inc.
(800) 285-4484

Wellbutrin
Glaxo Wellcome, Inc.
(800) 722-9294

Zoloft
Pfizer, Inc.
(800) 646-4455

Zyprexa
Eli Lilly & Co.
(800) 545-6962

INDEX

103338